A Field Guide to Bedside Ultrasound

by Shyr Chui and Meagan Moi

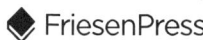 FriesenPress

Suite 300 - 990 Fort St
Victoria, BC, V8V 3K2
Canada

www.friesenpress.com

Copyright © 2016 by Shyr Chui and Meagan Moi
First Edition — 2016

The contents of this book remain the views and the opinions of the authors. Although the authors and publisher have made every effort to ensure that the information in the book was correct at the time of going to press, the authors do not assume and hereby disclaim any liability for loss, damage or disruption caused by errors or omissions, whether such errors or omissions result from negligence, accident, or any other cause. The contents of this book are not intended as a substitute for sound medical and clinical judgment by qualified physicians.

All images reproduced with permission.

All rights reserved. No part of this publication may be reproduced in any form, or by any means, electronic or mechanical, including photocopying, recording, or any information browsing, storage, or retrieval system, without permission in writing from FriesenPress.

ISBN
978-1-4602-9159-7 (Hardcover)
978-1-4602-9160-3 (Paperback)
978-1-4602-9161-0 (eBook)

1. MEDICAL, ALLIED HEALTH SERVICES, RADIOLOGICAL
& ULTRASOUND TECHNOLOGY

Distributed to the trade by The Ingram Book Company

Contents

Introduction 1

Chapter 1: Getting Started 5

Chapter 2: Doppler Ultrasound 9

Chapter 3: Scanning Conventions and Useful Terminology 15

Chapter 4: Saving, Storing and Reviewing Images 20

Chapter 5: Scrotum 25

Chapter 6: Abdomen 29

Chapter 7: Venous Doppler of the Leg 42

Chapter 8: The Female Pelvis 47

Chapter 9: Musculoskeletal and other applications 58

Chapter 10: Early Obstetrics (OB) 68

Chapter 11: Late Obstetrics (OB) 74

Chapter 12: Cardiac Sonography 78

Chapter 13: Ultrasound-Guided Procedures 89

Chapter 14: Choosing your new ultrasound machine 102

Chapter 15: Troubleshooting and FAQs 109

Afterword 114

List of abbreviations used in this book 116

Acknowledgements 118

References 119

About the Authors 121

Introduction

We are on the cusp of a revolution. Many would say the revolution is well underway. Over recent years, a combination of both the decreasing size and the increased affordability of ultrasound equipment has brought the use of ultrasound imaging out of radiology departments and closer to the point of care in emergency rooms, operating rooms, and intensive care units. The principle drivers have been the increased value ultrasound imaging can bring to clinical decision making at the point of care; and the increased confidence that ultrasound guidance can bring to interventional procedures.

In the near future, as ultrasound technology becomes more readily available, the reach of its clinical applications will extend further to the bedside, to examination rooms, and primary care clinics. In time, ultrasound units might become as important an aid to clinical examination as the stethoscope is today. Already, we see ultrasound skills being taught to the next generation of physicians in medical schools all over the world.

There is just one small problem. Using an ultrasound unit is difficult. The learning curve is somewhat long and shallow and hampered by the lack of experienced teachers "on the ground." Such educators have a vital role in providing students of this new art with critical feedback, not only on their technique, but also on the interpretation of their findings. The technology itself is complex to understand and the machines, although improving with every generation, have many knobs and buttons with unfamiliar labels. As a result, many users of point-of-care or bedside ultrasound find themselves limited at an early stage of their learning, limited to just a few clinical applications where they feel confident, and limited by their inability to develop their expertise as quickly as they would like. If this describes you and your situation, this book is for you.

This book is not for those who have progressed beyond that long, shallow part of the learning curve where a comprehensive text or atlas containing advanced knowledge might be more valuable. Similarly, this book has not been written for ultrasound technologists in training nor radiologists who may or may not be inclined to pick up a probe on occasion.

No, this book has been written for those who are just starting out on their ultrasound journey, who wish to take advantage of this amazing technology, to use it to aid their own practice, inform their clinical decisions, and guide their needles more safely.

You may ask why a radiologist and an ultrasound technologist would write this book in the first place? Not wishing to mix metaphors, the "turf war" over this technology between the radiology department and those beyond its walls has long been lost. The technology has escaped the radiology department. That ship has sailed and will never return. The question is no longer "who" should be using this technology but rather how can the medical community at large use ultrasound to provide timely, high-quality patient care, and improved patient outcomes? The short answer is with better education and that is the reason for writing this book. There is currently a great demand for simple, basic tuition on how to get started with bedside ultrasound, but the bulk of knowledge and expertise remains concentrated in the radiology department. Who better then to write this book than those who use this technology everyday, who are completely familiar with the machine, its controls, and the technique? Hence we are writing this book not only because we should but also because we can.

How should you the reader best approach this text? We have designed this Field Guide to be short, pocket sized, and available for quick reference. To achieve this, we have concentrated on mastering the machine and on basic probe handling technique. We have chosen to concentrate less on image interpretation and pathology, as this information is readily available elsewhere either in the form of online articles and larger texts, or in the expertise of regular users of ultrasound, be they a colleague, an emergency physician, a friendly radiologist, or technologist.

It should be emphasized from the outset, that sonographic findings should never replace or become a substitute for sound, clinical judgment. The overall, clinical assessment of the patient is paramount and sonographic findings only seek to augment, supplement, and inform this assessment and by doing so, enable more effective clinical decision-making and management.

In the first part of the book we will work through the basics including the principles of ultrasound and Doppler, scanning conventions, the most useful controls, and how to optimize your image. We have included a chapter on how to store and transmit both static images and cine clips for second review.

The second part concentrates on some of the more common applications you will likely encounter and the appropriate techniques required. These chapters include abdominal, pelvic, scrotal, lower limb venous, and early and late obstetrical ultrasound. We have also included a chapter on techniques for ultrasound-guided interventions. The chapters in this part of the book start with simpler scanning techniques, which gradually increase in complexity, thus complementing your increasing experience and degree of mastery of the technology. This culminates in a chapter on cardiac ultrasound and a simple technique to estimate left ventricular ejection fraction. In the interests of brevity, we have omitted many of the more advanced cardiovascular applications as well as intraluminal, endoscopic, and intravenous ultrasound for which separate, entire books could be written.

Dispersed throughout the book, we have included specific scanning tips, which we have discovered during our own learning and which will give your technique a little boost.

At the end of the book, we have included a chapter with practical advice on purchasing your first new machine and, because we all have those moments when nothing seems to go quite the way we expect, we have also provided a quick and practical troubleshooting guide, explaining what to do when the expected image doesn't appear on the screen when you think it should.

By now, I hope we have whetted your appetite enough to encourage you to read on and embark on your journey, probe in hand. Where should we begin? Let's start with the basics.

Chapter 1
Getting Started

The ultrasound unit is a complex machine with many components. In the interest of simplicity, we will describe here the basic controls that all units should have. The ultrasound unit is made up of a control panel with dials and controls for optimizing the image, as well as a keyboard for annotation. Some portable machines have a touch-screen display with all the controls available though different menus. There is a screen to visualize the structures being scanned, and of course there are multiple ultrasound probes that are used to create the image.

The basic premise of ultrasound is that the probes contain crystals which convert electric signals into high-frequency sound waves, defined as greater than 20 kHz. These sound waves travel into the patient, reflect off structures in the body and return to the camera to create a picture. Therefore, each pixel on the screen results from a returning sound wave. Why is this information relevant? Knowledge of the basic principles of ultrasound allows the user to interpret the images seen on the screen; that is different tissue types create different degrees of brightness on the image. For example, fluid-filled structures, such as the bladder or free fluid, appear black or *anechoic* on the ultrasound screen, whereas solid organs and soft tissues such as the liver, spleen, kidneys and uterus appear grey. Finally, dense tissues such as bone or calculi, are very bright or *echogenic* on the screen. However, one limitation of sound waves is they are impeded by air; therefore assessment of bowel is limited. The sound wave simply reflects off the air and the structures beneath are obscured by dark shadows.

Why do we need the Gel?

In order to create the image, we require coupling gel. This gel removes the air barrier between the skin and the probe, therefore allowing the sound waves to travel into the patient. Gel also acts as a lubricant, enabling the probe to glide easily on the patient's skin.

Types of Probes

There are three main types of ultrasound probe each with their crystals organized in different arrays that affect the shape and scope of the ultrasound beam produced. Different probes come with a variety of different frequencies, which not only affects the resolution but also the depth of penetration of the probe. The frequency and the penetration of the sound wave are inversely related to one another. Therefore a high-frequency probe has high resolution but low penetration, and the reverse is true for a low-frequency probe.

CURVILINEAR

This probe is rounded in shape, creating an arced face. Typically low in frequency, at about 5 MHz; this probe is optimal for assessing structures deep within the abdomen, such as liver, gallbladder, and pelvic organs. The rounded face of the probe creates a wide footprint, or *scope*, which allows larger areas to be assessed.

LINEAR

Rectangular in shape with a flat face, this probe comes typically in two frequencies: a medium frequency (6-8 MHz) optimal for vascular imaging, and a high frequency (12-18 MHz) optimal for small parts and musculoskeletal imaging. The high frequency linear probe has the better resolution, but sacrifices penetration and thus may not be able to visualize structures further away from the probe.

PHASED

Typically used in cardiac ultrasound imaging, or echocardiography, this low-frequency probe has a small rectangular footprint, but due to the arrangement of the crystals, creates an arced beam. The unique shape of this probe is optimal for assessing small spaces such as between the ribs.

Optimization of the Image

In addition to the dials discussed below, it should be noted that the correct scanning preset has a large impact on the quality of the image. The machine optimizes the image for each particular scan type, for example abdominal preset vs. pelvic or "gyne" preset. Always begin your study by selecting the correct probe and appropriate preset for the type of exam being performed.

DEPTH

This dial allows you to increase or decrease the depth of the sound wave generated. For example, by increasing the depth, you can image structures farther away from the probe such abdominal structures. Inversely, by decreasing the depth the image becomes more superficial, letting you optimize the image for structures closer to the probe.

FOCUS

By changing the position of the focus to the area of interest, the concentration of the beam is placed at the specified depth. For image optimization, we recommended you adjust the focus at or just below the level of interest. For example, when imaging the aorta, bring the focus down to the depth of the aorta.

GAIN

This control will either increase or decrease the brightness of the whole image, without increasing the amount of power applied to the patient. The gain of the image is very important, as maladjusted gain can impede the interpretation of the image. Aim to set the gain so that dark fluid-filled structures such as the bladder appear black but surrounding structures are still visible.

TGC (TIME GAIN COMPENSATION)

On the side of the ultrasound unit there will be a row of buttons on sliders. The sliders control the gain in the horizontal plane individually. These controls are particularly useful because they allow you to adjust the brightness at a particular depth, while leaving the rest of the image unaltered.

Chapter 2
Doppler Ultrasound

Introduction to Doppler

There are several different modes on the ultrasound unit. When ultrasound was initially developed, the probes utilized a single crystal and thus focused on the movement of a structure in the vertical plane. This mode is known as motion mode or *M-mode*. This mode is still used today in specific contexts such as measuring the fetal heart rate. Next, multi-array probes with hundreds of crystals were developed. These were able to interrogate multiple tissue structures in 2 dimensions creating brightness mode or *B-mode*. B-mode is the grey-scale image that we are familiar with today, as it displays the amplitude or brightness of each pixel.

In addition to these modes, the ultrasound unit is capable of detecting blood flow through the use of Doppler in three modes: color Doppler, power Doppler and spectral (or pulse wave) Doppler. A quick physics refresher is needed to understand how the ultrasound unit uses the Doppler effect to quantify blood flow. The Doppler effect is the shift in sound wave frequency created by a moving object. In this particular case, the moving objects are red blood cells. When the ultrasound beam emits a sound wave and then receives the reflected sound wave back from the moving blood cell, the unit calculates the difference in frequency. Depending on whether the frequency shift is increased or decreased, the unit interprets the difference as either a positive signal when moving towards the probe, or as a negative signal when moving away from the probe.

Color Doppler

Color Doppler interprets the changes in Doppler shift to create a color map of blood flow. Typically, the color map is a gradient of red to blue. Positive shift, when the blood is flowing towards the ultrasound probe, is reported as red in color and negative shift, moving away from the probe, is demonstrated as blue. There is a well-known mnemonic device to help you remember this: **BART B**lue **A**way **R**ed **T**owards. The velocity of the blood flow is represented qualitatively; fast velocities will be brighter in color, for example bright red/orange or light blue. Slow velocities will be dark red or blue, and finally, the absence of blood flow is depicted as black.

When you turn the color Doppler on, a small box will appear on the screen superimposing a color map over the 2D image. You can adjust the width and size of the color box and in addition, move the color box around the screen to assess particular structures. When using a linear probe, you can steer or angle the color box in different directions. When you turn the color box in the direction of the vessel, it becomes more sensitive to the Doppler shift. You can also increase the Color Doppler gain control as for B-mode. It is important to make sure that the gain is not set too low or you might miss blood flow. You can also adjust the scale (or velocity) of the color map. When you increase the scale, the maximum velocity displayable also increases on your image.

To make this even more confusing, there is a function on the ultrasound unit to reverse the color map, known as *invert*. This function is very handy as ultrasound protocol has developed such that when scanning blood vessels the color map is usually adjusted so that the arteries are red, and when scanning veins the vessels are usually imaged as blue.

Power Doppler

Power Doppler is similar to color Doppler, in that it also creates a color map to demonstrate vascularity. However, power Doppler is non-directional, instead detecting only the amplitude of the signal. Therefore, power Doppler is more sensitive to low-velocity flow, and is especially useful when assessing superficial structures or structures with low or trickle flow. Examples include slow-moving flow in calf veins or when assessing for torsion of the testis or ovary.

Spectral Doppler

Spectral Doppler refers to the use of a single ultrasound beam to detect the change in velocity of the Doppler shift. The resulting image creates a graph of blood flow and allows quantification of its velocity in a particular vessel. There are two types of spectral Doppler: pulse wave Doppler (PW) and continuous wave Doppler (CW).

PULSE WAVE (PW) DOPPLER

By using pulses of sound waves, the blood flow is interrogated at a specific depth and location. The cursor has a sample volume, and wherever this sample volume is placed, the blood flow at that specific location will be measured on pressing the "update" button.

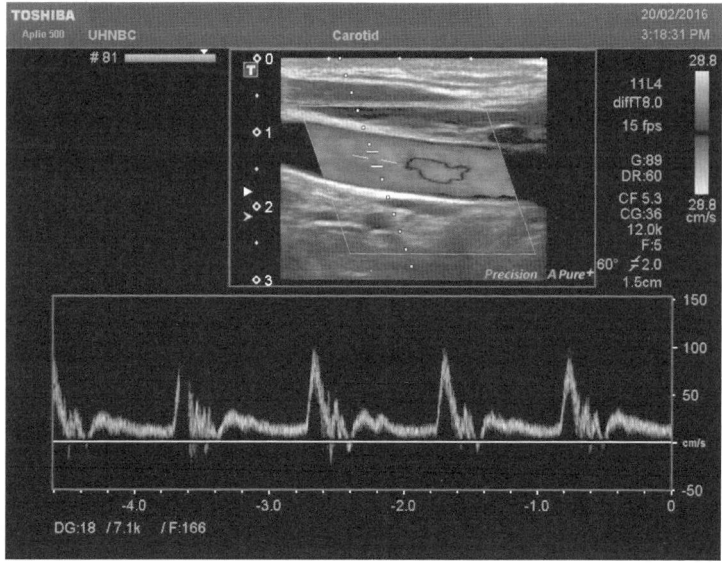

Figure 1. The above image shows a pulse wave sample of the carotid artery. At the top of the image the color Doppler box is seen with the pulse wave cursor. Below, the spectral trace of the velocity is shown.

CONTINUOUS WAVE (CW) DOPPLER

As the name suggests, this type of Doppler sends a continuous interrogation of sound waves through the entire beam. This type of Doppler is not depth specific, and therefore will display the highest velocity of the beam. CW is most commonly used in echocardiography.

Transmission Artefacts

There are several common artefacts seen on ultrasound that provide useful information about the characteristics of the structure being imaged.

POSTERIOR ENHANCEMENT

In a structure of low density, the sound beam accelerates through the structure and results in increased signals being interpreted deep to the structure. On the screen, this results in the area deep to this structure appearing brighter than the surrounding structures. A common example of this is a fluid-filled bladder, which appears anechoic. The sound beam is not attenuated as it passes through the bladder, which results in increased brightness and better visualization of the area deep to it. We take full advantage of this characteristic in pelvic imaging, where a full bladder provides an acoustic window to see the uterus and ovaries. Simple cysts, which appear as thin-walled, well-defined anechoic structures, will demonstrate the same properties.

POSTERIOR SHADOWING

When imaging high-density structures, such as bone or calcifications, the ultrasound beam is degraded and absorbed by these structures. The ultrasound unit interprets and displays this lack of returning signal as a black area deep to the dense structure. A prime example of this occurs when imaging gallstones. The stone will be echo bright with black shadowing posterior to it.

RING DOWN

Ring down is the term used for reverberation artefact. On the ultrasound image, ring down is displayed as a series of horizontal, linear lines, decreasing in width. Reverberation artefact occurs when two strong, sound-reflecting structures cause the sound beam to bounce between them. Ring down is commonly seen in the normal bladder, in bowel due to air, and in the gallbladder wall due to cholesterol deposits.

TWINKLE ARTEFACT

This color Doppler artefact occurs when assessing dense structures with color Doppler. It creates posterior "aliasing" or a flash of color. Twinkle is particularly useful when confirming the presence of calculi during assessment for renal stones.

Chapter 3
Scanning Conventions and Useful Terminology

In a similar way to conventional clinical examination of a patient, the ultrasound machine is usually positioned at the head and to the left of the bed and to the patient's right with the screen pointing towards the patient's feet. You, the operator would normally sit or stand on the same side of the bed facing towards the patient's head and directly facing the ultrasound machine's screen. If you are right-handed, this allows you to scan the patient with your dominant hand.

Every ultrasound probe has a small fixed marker at one end of the scanning surface. This marker corresponds to the end of the probe which generates the left side of the image on the screen. You can check this by gently touching the scanning surface of the probe at the marker end with your finger, and you should see some movement at the left edge of the screen image as you do this.

By convention, you should always orientate this probe marker and the left side of the image, either towards the patient's head or to the patient's right side during scanning. This also follows for any saved or printed images. If you hold the probe obliquely during scanning, the end with the marker should still be orientated towards the patient's head and right side as much as possible. This, in combination with accurate labeling of stored images, allows anyone reviewing your images to know the position of any imaged structure in relation to the long and short axes of the body. By always following this convention, you will develop the hand-eye coordination required for efficient scanning much more quickly.

You should hold the probe between your 4 fingers and thumb close to the transducer surface to allow greater fine motor control of the sound beam. As a rule, you should aim to protect your own elbow and shoulder from strain by positioning the patient as close to you as possible. When scanning the patient's left side, avoid reaching over and leaning across his or her body. This puts unnecessary strain on your arm, shoulder, and torso. Instead, ask the patient to roll up towards you halfway onto his or her right side. This is particularly important if you need to apply pressure with the probe to obtain a clearer image during obstetrical and abdominal scanning.

Always press the freeze button before you store an image. This makes it is easier to check its quality before you save it. Similarly, press freeze when you see your desired image and before you measure any on-screen structure with digital callipers. Before you store an image, annotate the image with the name of the structure or its location along with the relevant side of the body and whether the image is in the long axis, short axis, and sagittal or transverse plane. You will thank yourself later when you come to review the images.

Optimize the quality of your image at all times. Do this regularly during scanning. Some newer machines will do this with a single touch of the "auto image optimization" button. Even then, you will still need to adjust the depth to optimize the screen resolution to the target structure you are viewing. A common error is to have too much depth on screen, as this shrinks the target down to a small strip at the top of the image which you can barely see. If your machine does not have an auto-optimization feature, check your focus level matches the depth of the region of interest and adjust the gain accordingly.

When scanning, it is helpful to have a low level of ambient background light. Turn down the lights and draw the window blinds or curtains to achieve this and you will be able to see the screen image much more clearly. Most machines have illuminated controls for operation in low-light conditions.

Always respect the patient's privacy as much as possible. Close doors and draw cubicle curtains while you scan. Offer the patient an opportunity to change into a gown, if appropriate, to preserve their dignity. Ultrasound examinations usually require exposure of the patient's skin and may be intimate at times. When scanning sensitive areas, consider inviting a chaperone into the room for both your and the patient's peace of mind.

Useful Terminology

Three orthogonal body axes are used in medical imaging. These are the *sagittal*, *coronal* and *transverse (or axial)* planes. When using an oblique plane, it is named, by convention, to the closest of these three orthogonal planes, for example, *coronal-oblique*, *sagittal-oblique* or *transverse-oblique* planes.

Imaging planes and positioning

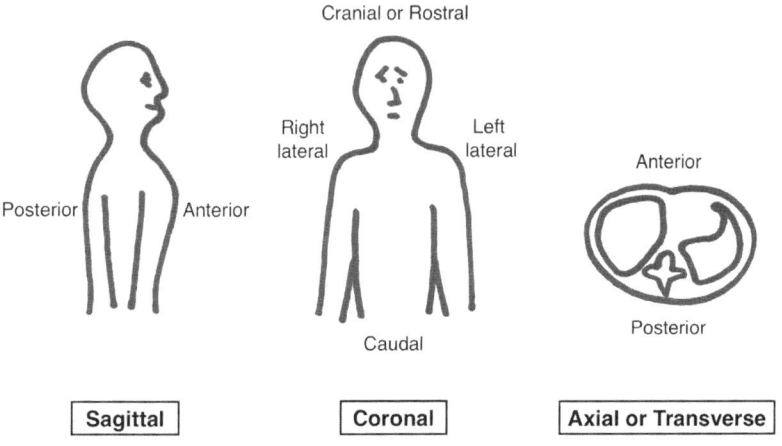

Figure 2. The three conventional scanning planes with associated terms for patient and probe positioning.

The relative positions within the body are depicted in Figure 2, *anterior* in front, *posterior* behind. *Cranial* or *rostral* is towards the head and *caudal* towards the feet. *Left* and *right lateral* are self-explanatory. These terms can also be used to denote direction in the body. Hence, *Antero-Posterior (AP)* means from front to back. *Cranio-Caudal (CC)* is from top to bottom.

The description of the brightness or darkness of a structure on the ultrasound screen is considered relative to the background level of brightness around that structure. Sound echoes generate ultrasound images and this is reflected in the terminology. Therefore, a structure, which appears dark relative to its surroundings, is termed *echo poor, hypoechoic,* or *hypoechogenic*. The opposite applies to relatively bright structures, which are termed *echobright, hyperechoic,* or *hyperechogenic*. If a structure is completely black and devoid of echoes such as a simple cyst, it is termed *anechoic*.

While the terms sagittal, coronal and transverse refer to the orthogonal axes of the body, any structure which has an oval, tubular, or eccentric shape, will have a *long axis* and *short axis* of its own which may be different from the true orthogonal axes. Hence, the gallbladder has its own long axis, which lies in an oblique-sagittal plane. The long axis of a kidney usually conforms to an oblique-coronal plane of the body.

The terms *superficial* and *deep* refer to their depth relative to the skin surface. *Linear* or *curved* are self-explanatory descriptors of a structure's shape. *Curvilinear* is a commonly used hybrid term.

Posterior acoustic enhancement, posterior acoustic shadowing and *ring down* artefact are terms described in the previous chapter on artefacts. *Artefacts* are artificially generated image abnormalities, which are often related to some physical manifestation of the imaging hardware or image-generating process.

The term *sound attenuation* refers to how much of the sound energy is absorbed by a structure, which subsequently alters the beam's propagation into the deeper tissues. If a structure such as fatty liver tissue demonstrates high sound attenuation, this will prevent visualization of the deeper part of the liver because insufficient sound energy penetrates through to the posterior liver for satisfactory image formation.

Doppler carries some additional terminology. *Hypervascular* and *hypovascular* are descriptors of blood flow and perfusion. *Augmentation* refers to an increase in blood flow in a vessel either induced manually by compressing the calf when assessing leg veins or induced physiologically during Valsalva manoeuvre.

Chapter 4
Saving, Storing and Reviewing Images

Any ultrasound study is a real-time examination. The most useful information is generated at the time of the scan itself, a dynamic process generating continuous images at the hand of the operator. Although the most useful and comprehensive information is gathered at the time of the study, it may nonetheless be valuable to review saved images or cine clips from a study after it has taken place. You should be aware however, that review of saved images and cine clips alone cannot provide the same level of information as the original real-time study. Saved images and cine clips can only provide "edited highlights" of the original study but are useful when you need a second opinion or if you intend to formally document your findings for the purposes of justifying a management decision. Sometimes, you may wish to keep images for educational purposes, perhaps to illustrate a talk, or solicit feedback from a mentor on your technique. In fact, in the absence of a teacher looking over your shoulder at the time of the scan, this timely solicitation of feedback is probably the next best way to learn ultrasound skills.

Saving images however, is a little more complicated than simply pressing the "store" button. When reviewed after completion of the study, ultrasound images of different parts of the body can be confusingly similar in appearance. Therefore, it is good practice to annotate your images with the name and side of the imaged body part. Ideally, you should include the orientation of the probe in your annotation: either long or short axis with respect to the organ, or sagittal or transverse relative to the axis of the body. Most machines will have some sort of text function for you to do this or a pictorial function where the probe orientation and position is displayed in the corner of the image. When scanning the breast, it is common practice to annotate an image of a focal abnormality by referencing the side, the position on the clock face relative to the nipple, and the distance from the nipple.

Tip

Most machines will automatically keep a record of the last few seconds of scanning when you push the freeze button. This can be accessed by "dialling back" with the trackball or using an on-screen "dial back" function. This is useful for reviewing and saving an image of something you might have passed over quickly.

In addition to image annotation, you should attribute the whole study itself to the correct patient by using patient identifiers such as the name, date of birth, and hospital or health numbers. You should do this at the start of the study before you select both the probe and study preset. The machine will generate a patient folder in the machine's disk directory into which images and cine clips can be stored and all of which, will be labeled with the patient's name. Changing the name after images are taken is not permitted on many machines to prevent mislabelling and misfiling of images into an incorrect patient folder. If you intend to save images for future review, we strongly recommend you take the few extra seconds required to input the patient details before you start the scan. Some point-of-care machines will save the images under a generic and automatically assigned, default case number individual to each case. This allows for image storage and review but the assigned case numbers are often long and complex and can be difficult to locate in the file directory at a later date, especially if many previous case studies have been stored in this way.

In a similar way, if you intend to transfer images to a patient's folder in an Electronic Medical Record (EMR) or in a Picture Archive and Communications System (PACS), you will need to ensure satisfactory registration of the patient's details on the machine with the EMR or PACS. Any difference in the patient's demographics between your ultrasound machine and these systems will cause a registration error and result in quarantining of the study until a broker can match the demographics, confirm the correct patient, and complete the transfer manually.

You can connect many ultrasound machines to thermal printers, which produce hard copy images. Providing patient demographics and annotating images is just as important with hard copy images, as the image is useless in the hands of another without these details. Hard copy images also present a potential privacy issue, as these can easily be removed, carried in a pocket, and accidentally lost in a busy emergency department.

Most machines allow you to record a short period of scanning by capturing cine clips, which you can review later as a mini movie. These are invaluable for capturing dynamic information such as the beating heart, flowing blood, or Doppler information. Cine capture can be either *prospective* or *retrospective* depending on your machine's set up. Many machines can capture in either mode but usually capture in one or the other. To acquire in *prospective* capture mode, *first* press the cine button, scan the requisite body part and then end the cine capture by re-pressing the cine button or freeze button. With *retrospective* cine capture, you should press the cine button *after* you have scanned the requisite body part and the machine automatically stores a pre-defined period of scanning prior to pressing the button. With *retrospective* cine capture, the length of this stored clip is usually set beforehand when the machine is bought and delivered. The vendor's applications specialist will help set up all your initial default settings and train you on how to use the machine. You can set the length of *retrospective* cine capture anywhere between a few seconds up to a minute, but you should bear in mind that longer clips use up more of the machine's hard drive memory per clip.

Tip
If you find yourself needing both hands to scan, perhaps one to hold the probe while the other augments venous flow by squeezing the calf, you can still save images for later review by using cine clip capture.

Reviewing stored images and cine clips is straightforward when they have been appropriately annotated. To review images, call up the patient directory, select the correct patient and press the "review images" button. This is a good time to obtain a second opinion and gain valuable educational feedback.

The only better way to learn is to have someone watch your scanning in real-time and give feedback there and then. If you are working alone or do not have someone immediately available, new live-streaming technology may be of value. Some machines come with this capability built in. If yours does not, there are several third-party solutions available which can link your machine to a secure network, over which a colleague or tertiary center specialist can watch your scanning live on a remote computer or device. They can offer not only a second opinion on the primary scan, but also real-time guidance on technique, positioning, and obtaining further views. Live-streaming technology is becoming increasing available and might completely transform how ultrasound imaging is both performed and interpreted in the future.

Chapter 5
Scrotum

Probe:

High-frequency linear

Preset:

Scrotum, Small Parts or Testis

Patient positioning:

Supine. Place a towel or ball of tissue behind scrotum and between legs to prevent testes falling out of view. Ask patient to hold penis up against the lower abdominal wall out of the way. Make sure the room is warm to prevent the testes retracting up into the inguinal canal.

Technique:

Apply gel. Ideally this should be warmed. Cold gel has the unfortunate effect of causing the testes to retract into the upper scrotum and away from view. Start in the short axis and image both testes in a single image to compare the echotexture and size of the two testes. If the field of view is too narrow to include both, switch to dual screen mode and match the transverse images of the left and right testes on the dual screens. Scan through both testes individually in long and short axis to look for a testicular mass or tumor. Apply color Doppler to assess and compare the perfusion of the two testes.

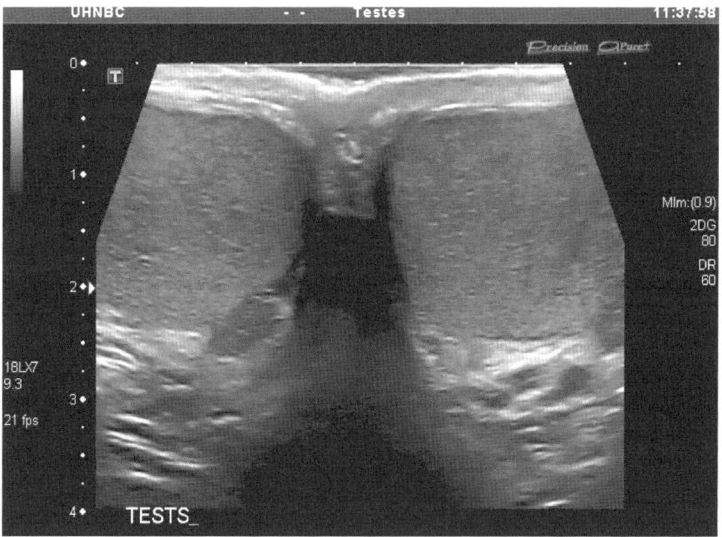

Figure 3. A transverse image of the left and right testes for comparison.

Tip

When assessing for torsion, apply color or power Doppler to the testis in question, turn the Doppler gain right up. All the vessels surrounding the testis will light right up like a fire but in complete torsion, the testis itself will remain dark with no perfusion.

Assess the epididymi looking for cysts, enlargement, and increased blood flow with color Doppler. With acute infection, the patient will often announce local tenderness during the ultrasound examination. Acute epididymitis usually starts at the tail with focal enlargement and increased perfusion relative to the asymptomatic side. Next, infection spreads to the entire epididymis and on to the testis (epididymo-orchitis). When infection is severe, look for an intrascrotal fluid collection or echogenic hydrocele indicating a potential developing intrascrotal abscess.

Assess for hydrocele (complex or simple) and for varicocele. A hydrocele, represented by anechoic fluid, usually extends almost completely around the testis. A large epididymal cyst however, usually lies to one side of the testis. A varicocele consists of dilated veins exceeding 3mm in diameter, which dilate further during Valsalva manoeuvre. Varicoceles typically extend inferior to the testis in the scrotum. If in doubt, apply color Doppler and the varicocele should light up with blood flow.

> **Tip**
> *In an older patient with a varicocele, switch to the curvilinear probe and using an abdomen preset, scan the kidneys. Tumor-thrombus from a renal carcinoma propagating into the left renal vein can result in a left-sided varicocele by occluding the distal testicular vein.*

If you are assessing for a scrotal mass, consider an inguinal hernia and extend the scan up into the inguinal canals, asking the patient to cough intermittently or strain down into the pelvis. Scanning the patient in the erect position will aid detection of a hernia.

Notes:

A full discussion of imaging in intermittent torsion will not be given here but bear in mind that with intermittent torsion, the testis can appear sonographically normal but the clinical presentation can be a precursor to complete testicular torsion.

Chapter 6
Abdomen

Probe:
Low-frequency curvilinear

Preset:
Abdomen

Patient positioning:
Initially patient supine

Prep:
Fasting, ideally for at least four hours, avoiding fatty foods prior to scan. This prep will distend gallbladder and reduce activity of bowel (which can impede visualization of organs).

Technique:

AORTA

Apply gel. Start with the aorta in the midline in the sagittal plane just above the umbilicus. If you encounter bowel gas, apply gentle but sustained pressure to displace gas and bowel loops away from beneath the probe. Angle the probe from side to side until you locate the pulsating aorta in long axis then scan along its length. The aorta bifurcates at the L3 lumbar level; so do not look for it below this level. Turn the probe 90° into the transverse plane and look for the aorta at its widest point. Measure the diameter with callipers from the leading edge of the wall to the opposite leading edge or estimate its size using the ruler at the side of the screen. Follow the aorta into the common iliac arteries to assess for iliac artery aneurysms. Apply color Doppler to assess for flow.

Tip

To distinguish the aorta from the inferior vena cava (IVC), look at the shape, the IVC is usually flatter with thin walls. Follow the vessel up towards the patient's head; the IVC passes through the liver, the aorta does not. Look for the major branches coming off the anterior abdominal aorta, the celiac trunk and the superior mesenteric arteries, which arise in close proximity to one another. Color Doppler will also help determine the direction of flow within the vessel.

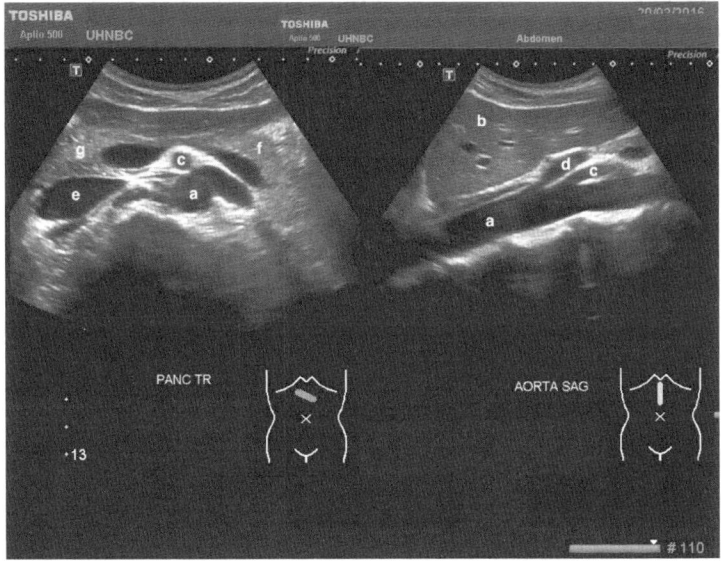

Figure 4. Dual screen image demonstrating a transverse view of the pancreas and sagittal view of the proximal aorta. On the right image, annotations indicate the proximal aorta (a) and left lobe of the liver (b). Branches of the aorta are seen including the superior mesenteric artery (c) and celiac axis (d). On the left image, the head of the pancreas (g) is seen anterior to the IVC (e). The pancreatic tail (f) is seen anterior to the aorta (a).

PANCREAS

Finding the pancreas can be difficult as it usually sits deep to multiple bowel loops and the stomach, which often contain gas. Start in the midline in the transverse plane and find the aorta and IVC at the midpoint between the sternum and the umbilicus, then gradually move the probe superiorly towards the patient's head. Sweep up and down looking for the splenic vein, a horizontal, black blood vessel above the aorta and IVC. The neck and the body of the pancreas can be found draped over the splenic vein. Angle the probe caudally to visualize the pancreatic head seen to the right of the splenic vein. Follow pancreatic tissue medially and deep to the superior mesenteric artery and vein (seen in transverse plane) to identify the uncinate process of the pancreas. Turn the probe into the sagittal plane to scan through the pancreatic head and uncinate process. You can often see the distal common bile duct if you angle away from the midline and to the right of the superior mesenteric vessels, now in long axis. The tail is often difficult to see due to bowel gas but you may get lucky if the patient is appropriately starved and you can displace the gas away with light pressure. The tip of the pancreatic tail is often best seen at the splenic hilum when assessing the spleen.

If you cannot see the pancreas at first, try applying gentle, sustained pressure with the probe to displace loops of bowel. Sometimes the pancreas is best seen in expiration. Don't spend too long looking for the pancreas. Even experts struggle with it at times. Come back later when the bowel gas might have moved on.

LIVER

Start in the midline in the sagittal plane at the upper abdomen just below the sternum. Look for the left lobe above the IVC. Sweep to the left, then turn 90° into transverse and sweep up and down through the entire left lobe. A liver tucked up under the ribs will be better visualized during deep inspiration. For the right lobe, turn and angle the probe obliquely upwards into the right upper quadrant and press down under the costal margin towards the right shoulder. Increase the depth and focus to include as much liver as possible, looking for the diaphragm at the deep and far side of the liver. Look for the IVC and hepatic veins draining into it. The diameter of the IVC and the degree of collapse during inspiration can be measured just below the diaphragm in the sagittal plane to assess for the patient's circulatory status. Scan up and down through the liver in sagittal and transverse planes. Sometimes, if the liver is tucked up high under the ribs, you will need to scan between the right lower ribs to see the right lobe. Find the portal vein on an oblique course at the liver hilum. Apply Doppler and look for the direction of blood flow. Look for dilated biliary ducts within the liver itself. The bile ducts follow the portal veins and look like dark tree branches when dilated. Bile ducts have no flow on application of color Doppler.

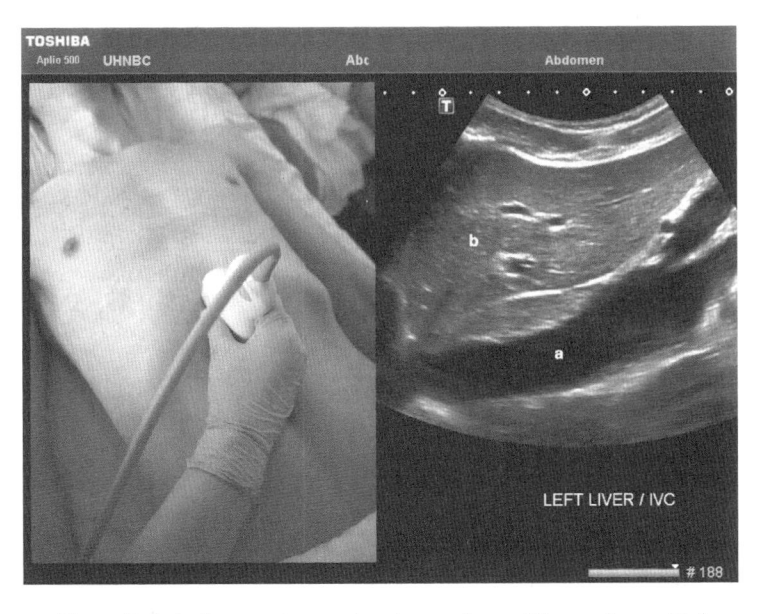

Figure 5. A dual screen image showing probe position and a sagittal image of the left lobe of the liver. The IVC (a) and the left lobe liver (b) are annotated.

Tip

A diffusely bright, echogenic liver usually denotes fatty infiltration (hepatic steatosis). In this condition, the echogenicity and brightness of the liver far exceeds that of the adjacent right kidney and attenuates the sound beam sufficiently to reduce visualization of the deeper, posterior right lobe of the liver. Geographical areas of reduced echogenicity in a fatty liver are often seen at the hilum or adjacent to the gallbladder bed. These can be confused with masses, but usually represent focal fatty sparing. With fatty sparing, the internal vasculature of the affected area appears normal on application of color Doppler, whereas a true hepatic mass will usually distort the normal pattern of hepatic vessels.

GALLBLADDER AND BILIARY SYSTEM

The gallbladder sits under the edge of the liver close to the junction of the left and right lobes, but its exact location can vary from patient to patient. Angling the probe at 45° should help you locate it. Once located, sweep though from fundus to neck, looking for echogenic stones casting posterior acoustic shadows. Gallstones can vary in size from a few millimeters to 2-3 centimeters. Measure the gallbladder wall on a short-axis image. Normal wall thickness should be up to 3mm. At the same time, you should assess for clinical tenderness as you scan directly over the gallbladder. Such focal tenderness is specific for acute cholecystitis, even with a normal thickness gallbladder wall. Ideally the patient should be starved for several hours before the examination for best visualization of the gallbladder. If they have recently eaten, the gallbladder might appear collapsed and be difficult to find. Sometimes the gallbladder appears contracted around multiple gallstones. Without the dark bile in the lumen, the gallbladder in this case will simply look like a curvilinear structure casting dense posterior acoustic shadows (Wall Echo Shadow or WES gallbladder) and can be misinterpreted as a loop of bowel. Complete evaluation of the biliary tree and gallbladder includes scanning the patient turned on their left side.

This often gives a better view of the gallbladder and also allows you to assess for mobility of any gallstones in the gallbladder lumen versus fixed stones lodged in the gallbladder neck. From the body of the gallbladder, scan towards the gallbladder neck. Turn the probe 90° so that the probe side marker now points towards the patients right shoulder, and look for the portal vein at the liver hilum. Locate the common bile duct (CBD) anterior to the larger portal vein. Look for the two structures running together in long axis and then look for the right hepatic artery in short axis as it cuts across between the portal vein and the CBD. The correct level to measure the CBD is at the level of the right hepatic artery. This view takes a lot of practice to master. Sometimes the right hepatic artery crosses anterior to the CBD, which is a normal anatomical variant.

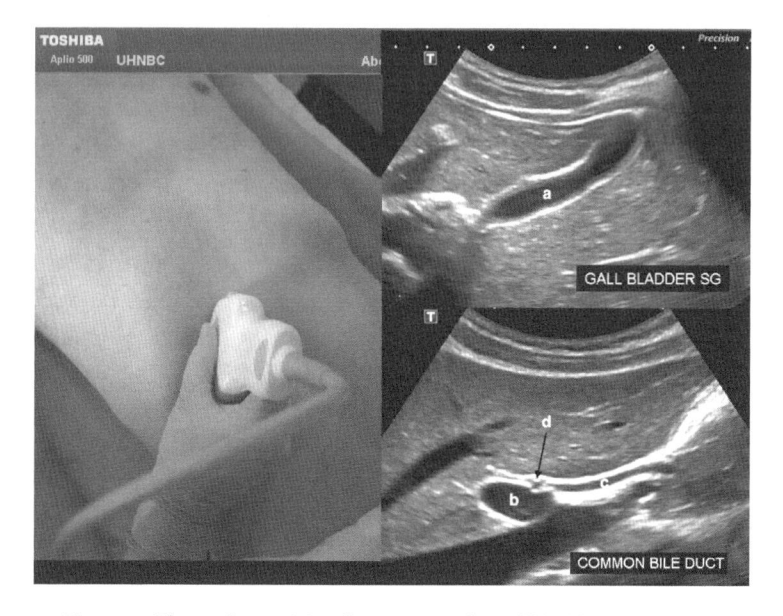

Figure 6. The probe position for imaging the gallbladder and CBD is shown above. The gallbladder (a) in the sagittal plane is demonstrated, and by turning probe 90° and sweeping laterally, the main portal vein (b) and the CBD (c) can be seen. The arrow (d) indicates the right hepatic artery, the level at which the CBD should be measured.

Tip

The normal diameter of the CBD should be 5mm or less but this increases with age. As a rule of thumb, after the age of 50 you can add a millimeter for every decade, so 6mm is normal in a 60 year-old, 7mm in a 70 year-old etc. After cholecystectomy surgery, an unobstructed CBD can appear larger and all bets are off.

KIDNEYS

Start with the right kidney, it's easier to find. Scan from the side of the patient in the coronal plane using the inferior right lobe of the liver as an acoustic window. Scan through the kidney in the long and short axis measuring the kidney at its longest dimension. Look for hydronephrosis, for echogenic calculi casting posterior acoustic shadows and for renal masses and cysts. It should be noted that small calculi might not cast posterior shadows. Cysts demonstrate posterior acoustic enhancement, whereas solid masses do not. With a cystic lesion, look closely for solid elements, calcifications and septations. If complex, apply color Doppler and look for internal perfusion. Solid lesions do not demonstrate posterior acoustic enhancement like cysts. Small, echogenic, solid masses can represent benign angiomyolipomas (AML) but also occasional early malignant tumors. Referring for follow-up CT imaging might be valuable in differentiating fat elements within these echogenic tumors and confirming an AML.

Tip

To differentiate isoechoic renal masses from prominent columns of normal renal cortex, use color or power Doppler. Normal renal tissue demonstrates a normal pattern of splaying vessels radiating from the hilum outwards. Tumors however, demonstrate irregular, multidirectional, internal vessels.

While assessing the kidneys, be sure to pass your ultrasound beam right through and beyond the renal borders in both long and short-axis planes. Otherwise, you could miss occasional tumors growing out from the very edge of the kidney. While assessing the right kidney, always check the hepato-renal (Morison's) pouch for dark free fluid. This is a common site for free intra-peritoneal fluid to pool in a supine patient.

Move to the left kidney. To save reaching over the patient, ask the patient to turn up halfway onto his or her right side.

Approach from a left lateral or posterolateral position. Often gas in the descending colon prevents a good view of the left kidney, so you might need to scan from a more posterior approach. Again scan through the entire kidney in both long and short axis evaluating as for the right side. If you are struggling to see the upper pole of the left kidney, try using the spleen as an acoustic window scanning through it to get to the kidney.

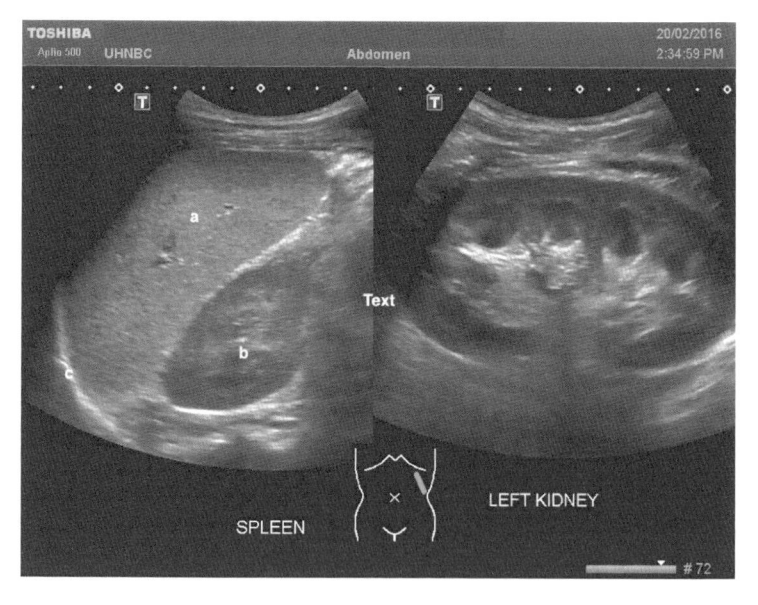

Figure 7. The dual screen image above shows the spleen (a) and the upper pole of the left kidney (b). The bright, curved structure seen superior to the spleen is the diaphragm (c). A long-axis image of the left kidney is demonstrated on the left image.

SPLEEN

Find the spleen above the left kidney under the left hemi-diaphragm. The spleen is best approached posteriorly and laterally. Measure the longest dimension for splenomegaly (13cm is the upper limit of normal) and assess for intra-splenic lesions. The spleen might be better assessed in expiration if the lower left lung obscures your view of the superior spleen.

FREE FLUID, COLLECTIONS AND HEMATOMAS

Scanning for free fluid in the four quadrants of the abdomen and pelvis is quick and easy. Free fluid is dark on ultrasound and pockets of free fluid are linear in shape or have sharp pointed corners and concave margins. This is in contrast to intraluminal fluid in bowel, which has convex margins and rounded edges with no sharp corners. Common locations for free fluid to collect are around the liver and spleen, below the liver, in the hepato-renal pouch, in the flank regions, around bowel loops in the left and right iliac fossae, and in the Pouch of Douglas (or cul-de-sac) in the midline lower pelvis.

Focal fluid collections such as abscesses and pseudo-cysts however, are more oval or rounded in shape and usually develop a definable, thin wall. The location of forming abscesses is usually related to either sites of recent surgery or bowel perforation, but will also develop at predictable sites depending on the anatomy of the peritoneal space; for example, abscesses around the liver and in the right flank region complicate right-sided colonic surgery.

Tip

Hematomas usually appear as well-defined, hypoechoic collections with some internal, low-level echoes when using a low-frequency curvilinear probe. If more superficially located, they will often demonstrate a linear pattern of internal echoes, but will not demonstrate any perfusion on application of color Doppler.

ABDOMINAL WALL

When assessing the abdominal wall for a mass or localized pain, switch to a higher-frequency probe. This will enable better visualization of the abdominal wall musculature for defects and hernias. Ask the patient to perform the Valsalva manoeuvre to help induce subtle, reducible hernias. Check for peristalsing bowel contents and manual reducibility. Apply Doppler to assess for strangulation. Look for masses in the abdominal wall and use Doppler to differentiate between hematoma and tumor.

APPENDIX

Ultrasound assessment of the appendix is difficult in adults and easier in children. Use the highest-frequency probe you can to maximize detail. Start at a point two-thirds along a line drawn between the umbilicus and the right anterior superior iliac spine (McBurney's point). Apply gentle, sustained pressure on the probe while being respectful of the patient's symptoms. Start in the sagittal plane and locate the ascending colon and cecum. This usually contains gas, has a coarse fold pattern, and descends in the right flank. Follow down to the tip of the cecum and look for a thin, blind-ending, non-peristalsing viscus extending from the tip of the cecum. This area might be tender and a little free fluid might be visible if the appendix is inflamed. The normal appendix is usually 6 millimeters or less in total thickness but secondary signs of tenderness and the presence of free fluid are important here. It should be noted that an appendix smaller than 6mm in diameter can still be acutely inflamed and an appendix larger than 6mm can be normal, hence secondary factors such as focal tenderness, localized fluid, lab results, and the overall clinical picture are more important than the absolute size of the appendix. Look for an echogenic appendolith in the lumen of the appendix, often seen in acute appendicitis. This usually casts a posterior acoustic shadow, different from the ring down artefact generated by gas in bowel. If the appendix descends into the pelvis or sits in a retrocecal location, it might remain unseen. If the appendix appears normal, look for enlarged mesenteric lymph nodes in the right iliac fossa or the midline, which might suggest alternate pathology such as mesenteric adenitis. Consider extending the scan to include the pelvic organs in women (see Chapter 8 Female Pelvis). Remember that ultrasound of the appendix is difficult but rewards the persistent learner and experienced operator.

BLADDER

The bladder can be found in the midline, lower abdomen just above the symphysis pubis and bony pelvic brim. Start in the transverse plane in the midline and scan down into the pelvis. A full bladder will appear as an anechoic, dark oval or round structure. Scan through it in both planes looking at its wall for focal lesions. If you see a mass arising from the bladder wall, apply color Doppler to distinguish a tumor from hematoma. Calculi cast dense, posterior acoustic shadows and sit posteriorly. In bladder outflow obstruction, the bladder can be huge and extend as far superior as the umbilicus.

Chapter 7
Venous Doppler of the Leg

Probe:
Medium-frequency linear or low-frequency curvilinear

Preset:
Leg Veins, Venous or DVT

Patient positioning:
Initially supine, then later sitting up with legs over the edge of the bed

Principles:
Ultrasonic assessment for deep vein thrombosis of the leg is straightforward but requires some prior knowledge of the expected anatomy and course of the deep veins. Normal veins have thin walls and the vein will collapse and compress when the operator applies pressure to it with the probe. The most accurate indicator of a patent vein completely free of thrombus is if the walls completely oppose one another during compression.

Color Doppler will demonstrate flow when the lumen is patent and during augmentation of flow induced by squeezing the thigh or calf below the level of examination. Partially occluded veins containing thrombus will also demonstrate some flow. An occluded and thrombosed vein will not compress and will demonstrate hypoechoic or isoechoic echoes within the vessel lumen. Acute thrombus usually appears hypoechoic, will expand the vein, and may be tender on pressure. Chronic thrombus is usually more echogenic, does not expand the vein, is non-tender, and might even partially recannalize in which case flow will return to the lumen.

Tip
If the thigh is large and the veins lie too deep for the medium-frequency linear probe, switch to the low-frequency curvilinear probe and narrow the sector width. This will maximize horizontal resolution by concentrating the same number of sound generating crystals within a narrower sector but at the same time allow for greater depth of penetration by virtue of its lower frequency.

Technique:

Apply gel. Start with the patient supine at his or her groin just below the inguinal ligament. With the probe in transverse, locate the Common Femoral artery and vein as two oval black structures. Closer examination will reveal the thicker wall, rounder shape, and pulsatile appearance of the artery. Apply downwards pressure on the vessel using the probe in your hand. The vein, if patent, will compress but the artery will not and the pulsatile appearance of the artery will become more prominent. Moving caudally, apply intermittent compression every 2-3 centimeters whilst looking for the patent "winking vein." Watch the artery bifurcate into the Superficial and Profunda Femoral arteries. The more superficially located Long Saphenous vein will arise from the Common Femoral vein anteriorly in the groin, before continuing down the medial aspect of the leg close to the skin. Proceed down the thigh following the Superficial Femoral vein, compressing intermittently to check for venous patency.

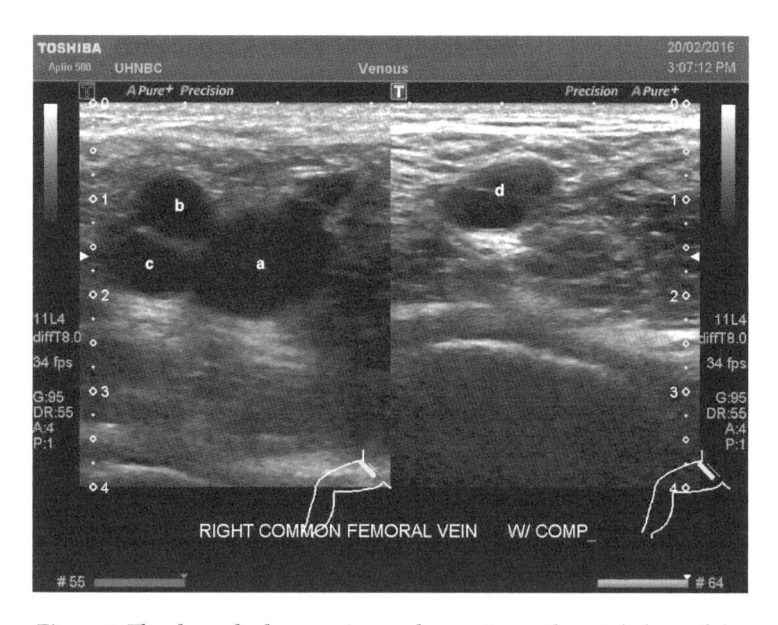

Figure 8. The above dual-screen image demonstrates the axial plane of the Common Femoral vein, uncompressed and with compression. Indicated on the left, is the Common Femoral vein (a), Superficial Femoral artery (b) and Profunda Femoral artery (c). On the right, with compression, the arteries (d) remain visible while the vein has collapsed.

Tip

In the lower medial thigh, the Superficial Femoral vein and artery dive deep to a tough connective tissue layer in the "adductor canal." Compression from above becomes difficult and painful. Instead, keep the probe over the vein and artery but place your other hand under the patient's thigh and pull the whole thigh upwards against the probe. The vein will still "wink" at you if patent.

For the Popliteal and calf veins, sit the patient up on the edge of the bed dangling both legs over the edge. Gravity will increase venous distension and help you see them. Ask the patient to shuffle forward a little so that you can get your probe behind his or her knee. Scan in transverse behind the knee looking for the popliteal artery and vein. Usually the vein in this position lies closer to the probe than the artery. Compress the Popliteal vein to check for patency. While in this position look for a Baker's cyst in the medial popliteal fossa. A Baker's cyst is a thin-walled fluid collection arising from the posterior knee-joint capsule with its neck extending between the medial head of gastrocnemius tendon and the semimembranosus tendon. When you see a Baker's cyst, check for any internal echoes suggesting potential internal hemorrhage or for dark, linear fluid around the Baker's cyst (perhaps extending down the calf), which might suggest recent rupture.

In the calf, continue down the posterior calf in the midline. Watch the Popliteal vein split into the paired, peroneal deep stem veins, which usually flank the peroneal artery. Compression applied here will result in the paired veins "blinking" at you on either side of the artery if patent.

You can see the Posterior Tibial deep stem veins more medially in the calf. Identify them first in the lower calf above the ankle and then follow them upwards towards the knee and popliteal vein. Again compression of the paired Posterior Tibial veins results in "blinking" veins either side of the Posterior Tibial artery when patent. As you reach the upper calf, the Posterior Tibial veins dive deep to muscles, where compression can be difficult and painful but persist nonetheless to demonstrate venous patency. In the upper calf, you can also see the deep intramuscular gastrocnemius veins as they feed into the popliteal vein. Early thrombus may hide in these veins which will not compress if thrombosed. In circumstances where views are poor, use color Doppler to assist you. Use an angled color Doppler box (parallelogram shaped) when scanning along the long axis of the vein and a square or rectangular box when scanning in the vein in short axis. Using the correct box shape always increases the equipment's sensitivity to blood flow. It can be helpful to augment flow by squeezing the calf or thigh below the level of examination, but remember that partially thrombosed veins can still demonstrate some flow. Reduce the color Doppler scale, if necessary, to increase sensitivity for low-velocity flow.

The Anterior Tibial deep stem veins are small and rarely contain significant thrombus. These can be visualized by scanning from an anterior approach between the tibia and fibula. The small, paired Anterior Tibial veins run close and anterior to the interosseous membrane between the tibia and fibula and again, flank the Anterior Tibial artery on either side. When patent, these veins will again compress completely and appear to "blink" at you.

Tip

Occasionally, you will encounter normal anatomical variants. The commonest is duplication of the Superficial Femoral vein in the thigh and in this case, it is important to follow both duplicated veins as either one or both might contain thrombus.

Chapter 8
The Female Pelvis

Probe:

Low-frequency curvilinear

Preset:

Pelvic or Gyne

Positioning:

Supine. Ask the patient to lower pants to below the pubic bone.

Prep:

A full bladder is essential to transabdominal pelvic ultrasound scan. Have the patient fill their bladder by drinking 1 litre of water beforehand.

Technique:

The female pelvis can be imaged through two main sonographic techniques: transabdominal scanning, using the full bladder as an acoustic window, and transvaginal scanning, using a specific transvaginal ultrasound probe that is inserted into the vaginal canal.

Transabdominal Scanning

THE UTERUS

Apply gel to the probe and place on patient's lower abdomen, just above the pubic bone. Begin with the probe in the sagittal position. Provided that the patient's bladder is properly filled, you will see a dark structure that represents the fluid-filled bladder. A full bladder is an important tool for assessing the pelvis, as it creates a window by moving bowel out of the way and pushing the uterus flat. Without a full bladder, visualization of the uterus and ovaries is very difficult and limited. If the patient is unable to fill her bladder, consider transvaginal scanning. The uterus is a pear-shaped organ. In the sagittal plane, the uterus lies horizontally on the screen with the dome or "fundus" of the uterus lying superiorly towards the top of the image and the cervix inferiorly. Within the uterus, running from the cervix to the fundus, you will see an echo-bright stripe, representing the endometrium.

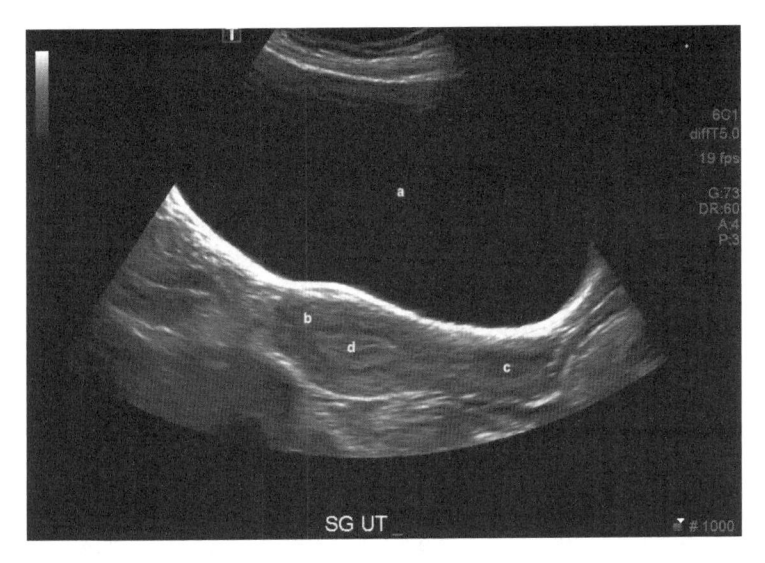

Figure 9. The above sagittal image demonstrates the uterus as seen transabdominally. Indicated are the fluid-filled bladder (a), the fundus of the uterus (b), the cervix (c), and the endometrium (d).

Tip

The uterus can lie in any orientation within the pelvis. Best visualization of the uterus occurs when the uterus lays anteverted i.e. pointed anteriorly. However, another common position is retroverted, when the uterus is tipped posteriorly. In this case, transvaginal ultrasound provides optimal assessment of the uterus.

Turn the probe 90° to the transverse position and starting low down, sweep upwards from the cervix to the fundus. When viewing the uterus in transverse, it appears as a circular structure. As you angle the probe towards the patient's feet, you will see a circular structure with two shadows posteriorly. This represents the cervix. Scan towards the patient's head. As you sweep upwards, you will move into the lower uterine segment and then into the fundus of the uterus. At the level of the fundus, the uterus appears circular in shape with the endometrial stripe in the middle. The endometrium varies in appearance depending on the patient's age and stage of menstrual cycle. It is always useful to determine the first day of the patient's last menstrual cycle to correlate with the endometrial appearance.

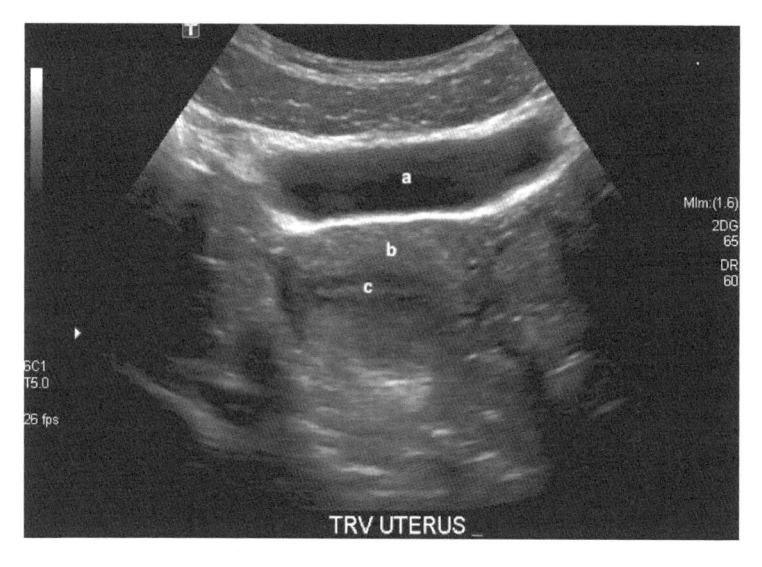

Figure 10. In the transverse image of the uterus, at the level of the fundus, the fluid filled bladder (a) is seen. Posterior to the bladder, the body of the uterus (b) and the endometrium (c) are indicated.

Tip

If you see a bright, linear object, generating ring-down artefact within the endometrial canal, ask your patient if they have an intrauterine contraceptive device such as a Copper T or Mirena

In reproductive-aged women, the endometrium ranges from thin, early in the menstrual cycle, a triple lined appearance mid cycle, and thick in late cycle. In the postmenopausal patient population, the endometrium should be thin and less than 5 millimeters. Women on hormone replacement therapy are the exception, in which case a maximal diameter of 7 mm is acceptable.

Tip

In the post-partum patient, the uterus will appear enlarged and the endometrium might be thickened. However, take special care to assess for blood flow within the endometrium. If present, this might represent retained products of conception, especially if the patient presents with per vaginal bleeding.

OVARIES

The ovaries lie adjacent to the uterus in the pelvis in the right and left lower quadrants respectively. Often, it can be challenging to locate the ovaries, especially in the postmenopausal patient population, as they shrink with age and can be hidden by adjacent bowel. To locate the ovary, start with the probe in transverse position low in the pelvis, angle upwards and slightly oblique. Ovaries are oval in shape, often described as "almond shaped," are echo bright and contain multiple, dark spots which represent the follicles. Sweep superiorly and inferiorly through the ovary in transverse. Carefully rotate the probe 90°, so that the probe is now sagittal, and again sweep right to left through the ovary. Once you have located an ovary, sweep through it to assess for masses or cysts. Fluid-filled cysts appear as dark, round, well-defined structures, with posterior enhancement. Ovarian masses may have a variable appearance, typically heterogeneous in echotexture, irregular in shape, and demonstrating internal blood flow when you apply color Doppler.

Similar to the endometrium, the ovaries also have a variable appearance dependent on the stage of the menstrual cycle. Early in the menstrual cycle, there are many anechoic follicles present within the ovary. Mid cycle, just before ovulation, a dominant follicle might be seen, represented by a round, anechoic structure. Finally in late cycle, you will see the collapsed remnant of the follicle as the corpus luteum. Typically, the corpus luteum will appear as an echo-poor, circular lesion with a thick wall and peripheral perfusion on application of color Doppler.

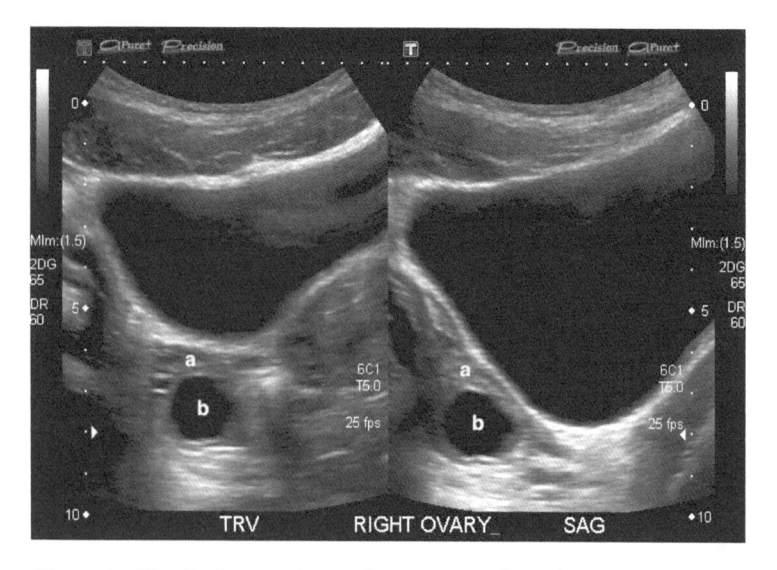

Figure 11. The dual-screen image demonstrates the right ovary in the sagittal and transverse planes. As shown, the ovarian tissue (a) is echogenic and in this patient, there is a dominant follicle (b) present.

It should also be noted that in the female pelvis, the presence of a trace of free fluid is normal. The best locations to find free fluid are posterior to the uterus, in the Pouch of Douglas, or anterior to the uterus in the anterior cul-de-sac. Free fluid might also be seen in the adnexae adjacent to the ovaries.

Transvaginal Ultrasound

Transvaginal ultrasound is a useful tool when transabdominal pelvic scanning is limited. However, transvaginal ultrasound is an advanced technique and can be difficult for beginners. It should be noted that this is an invasive procedure and should only be undertaken when indicated. We should stress that the transvaginal probe must be properly sterilized before every use. Most emergency departments have an established endocavity sterilization protocol, and it is absolutely crucial that the user is familiar with the process for probe sterilization before attempting to perform transvaginal ultrasound. The probe also requires the application of a sterile condom before use with each patient.

The transvaginal probe is a high-frequency probe and therefore the resolution of the images is significantly improved when compared to transabdominal scanning. However, due to its higher frequency, the field of depth is limited. Position the patient supine, with a bolster underneath the hips to elevate the pelvis and with knees bent. If the patient is lying on a gynecological stretcher, the use of stirrups might be appropriate. First apply gel to the probe transducer surface before fitting the probe cover or condom. Next apply sterile gel to the end of the covered probe to remove air between the probe and the pelvic structures.

Tip

Plug the endocavity probe into the ultrasound unit before beginning transvaginal scanning. This way, if you encounter air artefact, you can rectify this before inserting the probe into the patient.

Insert the transvaginal probe into the vaginal canal and rest it at the fornix of the cervix. The image seen from with transvaginal ultrasound has a slightly different orientation compared to a transabdominal study and it can require some practice to become familiar with the anatomy. Due to the location of the camera and when scanning in the sagittal plane, the cervix is seen at the top of the image right next to the transducer surface. The bottom of the image will be towards the patient's head and the uterine body and fundus will be seen here. Provided that the uterus is lying in an anteverted position, the right-hand and left-hand sides of the image represent the anterior and posterior aspects of the uterus respectively. By sweeping the camera from right to left in the sagittal plane, you can assess the whole uterus and adnexae.

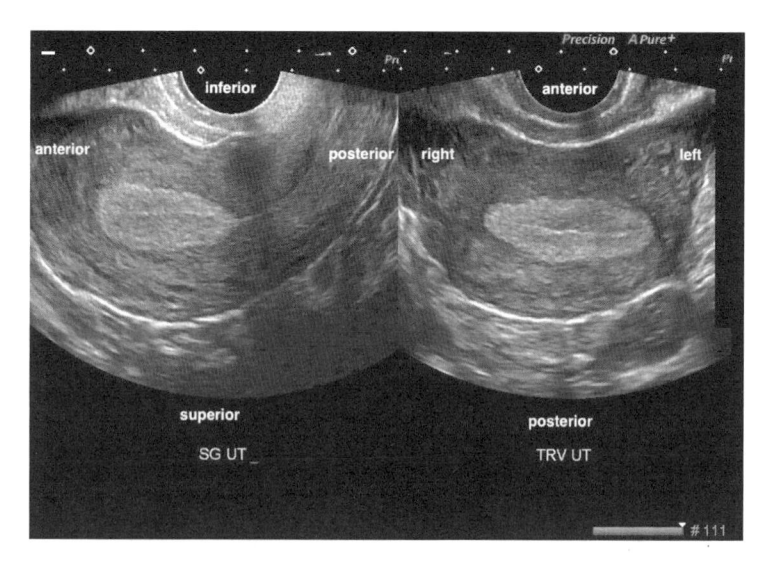

Figure 12. Transvaginal image of the uterus is demonstrated in the image above. As shown by the annotations, the scanning planes differ from conventional transabdominal scanning.

Tip

If you are having difficulty assessing the fundus, ask the patient to raise her hips for a moment, as this allows more room for angulation of the probe.

By turning the probe 90° so that the indicator on the probe is facing the patient's right side, you can assess the uterus in short axis. To scan inferiorly towards the cervix, raise the handle of the probe and angle it downwards. This allows you to visualize superior uterine structures such as the body of the uterus and the fundus. By lowering the handle of the probe and angling upwards whilst maintaining a transverse scanning plane, the uterus appears as a circular structure with the endometrium at the centre.

Tip

Many reproductive-aged women have a fibroid uterus and these benign masses can impede assessment of the uterus tissue and ovaries. Fibroids appear as hypoechoic, solid lesions within the uterus and are accompanied by a shadowing artefact. Look for any fibroids that distort the endometrial cavity, as these might be responsible for severe menorrhagia symptoms.

To assess the ovaries, start in the sagittal plane and angle the probe to the side of interest. Sweep laterally towards the iliac vessels. Often the ovary lies adjacent to the iliac vessels, which are an excellent landmark for ovary visualization. If the ovary is not seen, turn into the transverse plane while still in the lateral position, and sweep the probe anteriorly and posteriorly in the patient. Ovaries may be difficult to locate even with transvaginal ultrasound, and especially if the bowel is very active or if the ovary is sitting outside the field of view.

Tip
Bowel loops often prevent visualization of the ovaries. To move bowel out of the way, try pressing firmly on the patient's lower abdomen with your free hand, as this will sometimes displace the bowel and reveal the ovaries.

Acute Pelvic Pain

OVARIAN CYSTS

Ovarian cysts are a common pathology responsible for acute pelvic pain especially in the reproductive-aged patient. Ovarian cysts can have a variable appearance depending on the characteristics of the cyst. By definition, a simple cyst will appear as a round, anechoic structure with posterior enhancement, located within the ovary, and containing no internal blood flow on color Doppler. Cysts with septations or with internal bleeding have a more complex appearance on ultrasound. For example, a hemorrhagic cyst has a complex appearance with low-level, internal echoes and no internal flow on color Doppler, but will still be thin-walled, round, and well defined.

Tip
Is it a dominant follicle or an ovarian cyst? A dominant follicle has the same appearance as a simple cyst. In order to be classified as a cyst, and not a physiologically normal follicle, the cyst must be greater than 2.5 cm.

Be on the lookout for large amounts of anechoic free fluid within the pelvis, especially in the Pouch of Douglas or in the adnexa. This might represent an ovarian cyst that has ruptured, a potential cause for acute pelvic pain. The presence of a large cyst or mass, especially in a patient presenting with severe, acute-onset pelvic pain, can raise concern for ovarian torsion. A torsed ovary on ultrasound has a distinctive appearance; it is enlarged, often very round in shape, and has no internal blood flow. When ovarian torsion is suspected, we recommend the use of both color and power Doppler to confirm that there is no blood flow within the ovary. Be aware that ovarian torsion is a medical emergency and requires immediate action.

Chapter 9
Musculoskeletal and other applications

This chapter covers some additional applications of bedside ultrasound not included in the other chapters, but which are commonly encountered in emergency rooms or similar acute scenarios. This chapter is not designed to be comprehensive in breadth but outlines some of the more common applications.

Musculoskeletal (MSK)

PROBE:
High or medium frequency linear

PRESET:
MSK

PATIENT POSITIONING:
Variable, but allow room for dynamic imaging with both passive and active movement at a joint.

TECHNIQUE:
MSK ultrasound may seem straightforward but is surprisingly difficult to perform well and consistently. A thorough understanding of the relevant normal anatomy is key. Some parts are

easier to scan than others. The Achilles, quadriceps, and patellar tendons are straightforward. The rotator cuff, elbow or ankle are much more complex and require extensive scanning experience and more formal training which is beyond the scope of this book.

In capable hands, ultrasound imaging can evaluate tendons, muscles, ligaments, joints, synovium, and to an extent, bony structures for fractures and erosions. For the purposes of those starting out with ultrasound, we shall confine this discussion to the larger superficial tendons such as the Achilles, quadriceps, and patellar tendons.

Normal tendons have a specific, sonographic appearance. Their fibrillar structure is well seen in detail, appearing striped when viewed in long axis and spotted in short axis. When disrupted, the tendon fibers become discontinuous and interspersed with dark fluid, and hemorrhage. When acutely torn or chronically inflamed, the tendon also loses its thin, uniform shape, instead becoming expanded and fusiform in appearance. Tendon tears can be partial or full thickness in type. When a normal tendon is imaged at 90° perpendicular to the sound beam, the fibers are well seen, but if imaged even at a slight angle away from 90°, the normal fibrillar appearance is lost due to an artefactual phenomenon called *anisotropy*. When the probe is returned to a 90° angle relative to the tendon, the linear fiber pattern reappears. This anisotropy effect often causes diagnostic difficulty in distinguishing normal tendon from tears and tendon pathology, especially when tendons curve over underlying structures such as bones and joints and particularly at their bony insertions. You must be careful therefore, to maintain a 90° angle between the probe and tendon as much as possible.

> **Tip**
>
> *When scanning superficial structures such as tendons or joints, the curved nature of the structure under evaluation often prevents getting good probe to skin contact along the whole length of the probe's scanning surface. In this case apply a "gel pad", a large, thick blob of contact gel, over the region of interest. This allows the probe to stand off the skin slightly but still maintain good sound contact through the gel.*

A dark, fluid-filled, full-thickness tendon gap between the torn ends of a tendon makes the diagnosis of a complete tear easy. Sometimes, you might not see a gap but rather a dark, expanded tendon with loss of the expected internal fiber structure. In this scenario, it can be difficult to distinguish between a partial or complete tear. A big advantage ultrasound has over the other imaging modalities, such as CT or MRI, is its ability to image in real time while moving the joint or tendon. When a tendon is completely torn and the joint moved passively to stretch the tendon, the distal part of the tendon attached to the bone will move with the bone, but the proximal part above a complete tear will not. With partial tears, both proximal and distal ends will move together as some fibers remain intact. This dynamic evaluation is invaluable and applies to any potentially torn tendon from the smallest in the finger to the largest at the knee.

Therefore, when scanning the quadriceps tendon superior to the patella or the patellar tendon inferior, flex the knee joint to stretch the tendon and assess for a complete tear in this way. When assessing the Achilles tendon, dorsiflex the ankle slightly to assess for complete vs. partial thickness tear.

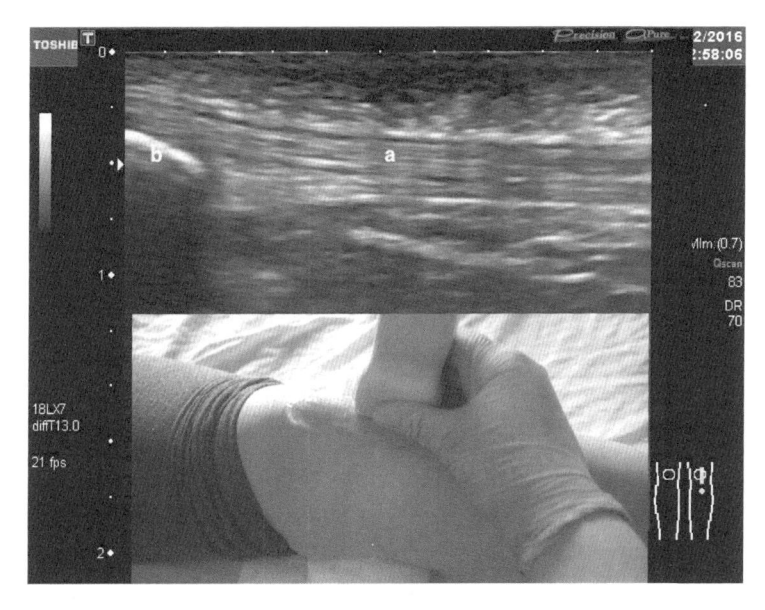

Figure 13. The probe position for scanning the patellar tendon is shown with the patellar tendon (a) in the sagittal plane as recognized by its fibrillar pattern. The echobright structure superior to the tendon represents the patella (b).

From a positioning point of view, when scanning the quadriceps and patellar tendons, have the patient lay supine. Roll up a towel and place it under the knee to flex the knee slightly and place both tendons under slight tension. This will straighten out the tendons and help you to see the linear fibrillar structure better. It will also open up any tendon gap slightly increasing the chances of spotting a tear if present. Scan in both the short and long axis of the tendon. Look for tendon discontinuity or fiber disruption and hematoma. Scan the asymptomatic, contralateral side for comparison if you are unsure of your findings and don't forget to add dynamic testing to differentiate between complete and partial tears. Don't forget to look at the cortex of the patella for a potential fracture line and cortical disruption.

For the Achilles tendon, lay the patient prone and place a towel under the front of the ankle or dangle the foot over the end of the bed. Scan in both long and short axis and compare with the contralateral side. Achilles tendon tears usually occur 4-7 cm above the calcaneal insertion at a relatively avascular zone of the tendon. Dynamic imaging here is also extremely useful.

Tip
In the absence of a history of trauma, a thickened, dark tendon with loss of the normal fiber pattern is likely to reflect chronic tendon pathology such as tendinosis. In this case you might see focal, round or linear, echobright calcifications in the tendon. On application of color Doppler, you might see blood flow in small vessels within the tendon. Normal tendons do not demonstrate vascularity like this and such "neovascularization" is indicative of a chronic healing response in a damaged tendon.

Lung

PROBE:
High-frequency linear or curvilinear

PRESET:
"Superficial" or "small parts"

PATIENT POSITIONING:
Supine for pneumothorax, erect or semi erect for pleural effusion.

TECHNIQUE:
Normal lung is poorly seen with ultrasound as the air within the lung parenchyma does not transmit and reflect sound in a

useful way. The air at the surface of the lung however, appears as a thin, bright line below which only "ring down" artefact can be seen.

During normal breathing, the surface of the lung moves appropriately as the lung expands and contracts. Lack of such movement indicates pneumothorax because air in the pleural space does not move with breathing. For optimal detection of pneumothorax, position the probe at the front or at the side of the chest over and between the ribs. Some users advocate the use of M-mode imaging to help confirm the movement of the air in aerated lung with breathing[1].

Consolidated lung is seen well with ultrasound, and consolidated lung has a similar appearance to the liver, but clearly lies above the echogenic, curvilinear diaphragm. Air bronchograms in consolidated lung appear as thin, branching, echogenic foci demonstrating "ring down" artefact. Pleural fluid is easy to see, appearing black and usually in a dependent location. With moderate to large pleural effusions, there is usually some collapse of the underlying lung, in which case the collapsed lung parenchyma might adopt a solid, triangular or curvilinear appearance.

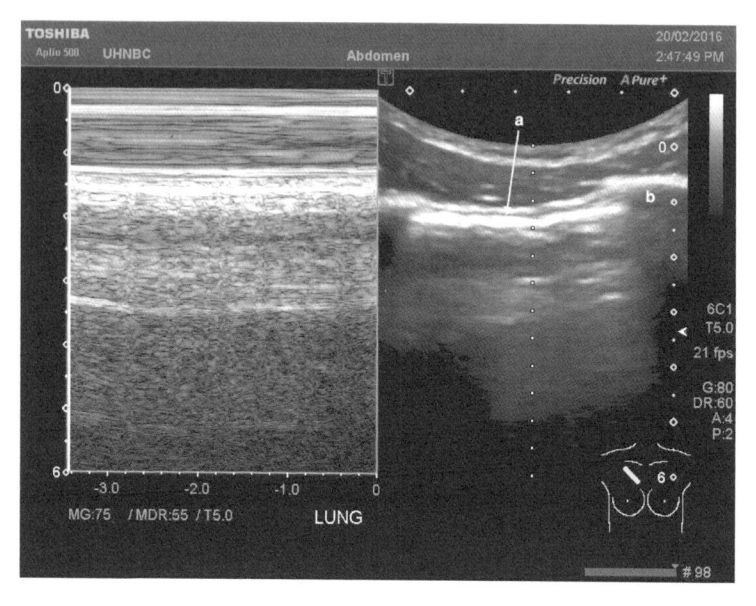

Figure 14. The following image demonstrates intercostal ultrasound of the pleura (a). On the right image, the echogenic line represents the pleura (a) while (b) represents the rib with posterior shadowing. On the left image, a M-mode trace demonstrates the "seashore" sign of normal pleural motion[1].

When looking for a pleural effusion, you should ask the patient to sit up and lean forward (if they are able) and then scan from a posterior approach. This allows gravity to pool the pleural fluid in the lower chest, aiding its detection. This is also a good position for needle aspiration of the fluid if required (see Chapter 13 Ultrasound-guided procedures). In a supine patient, anechoic, pleural fluid can be seen in the lower chest above the diaphragm when scanning the abdomen in the left and right upper quadrants.

Subcutaneous Foreign Bodies

PROBE:
High-frequency linear

PRESET:
"Superficial" or "Small parts"

PATIENT POSITIONING:
As appropriate for accessing the region of interest

TECHNIQUE:
Foreign bodies are a common complaint in the emergency room. Appropriate history from the patient is usually forthcoming as to the material, size, and location of the suspected foreign body, which you are seeking to locate.

Place gel around the puncture site. Use sterile gel if the wound is open. Start at the puncture site and work outwards. Set your focal zone indicator very superficially to maximize detection. Scan in both sagittal and transverse planes. Foreign bodies of any material will usually (but not always) have a bright, linear appearance, extending obliquely and deep from the puncture site. Most will also cast a posterior acoustic shadow behind them. Gravel will appear more focal and again bright with dense posterior acoustic shadows. You can improve sonographic visualization of linear foreign bodies, if the sound beam is at 90° to the object in question. You can achieve this by tilting or rocking the probe, also known as "heel-toe" positioning.

Ocular Ultrasound

PROBE:
High-frequency linear

PRESET:
"Superficial", MSK or "small parts"

PATIENT POSITIONING:
Supine, eyes closed.

TECHNIQUE:
This is a specialist application but nonetheless useful in certain circumstances. In the case of trauma to the eye or when clouding or hemorrhage in the anterior or posterior chamber prevents direct, ophthalmoscopic evaluation, you can use ultrasound to evaluate the lens, ciliary body, retina, optic nerve, sclera, and posterior globe. Use the high-frequency linear probe and a "small parts" preset. Lay the patient down in a supine position. Apply copious amounts of gel to the skin surface of the closed eyelid and scan through the eyelid. It is important not to apply too much pressure. To avoid this, hold the probe close to the transducer surface between your thumb, index and middle finger tips and rest the side of your palm down gently on the side of the patients face to stabilize the probe. This will allow small and precise movements of the probe. Scan straight downwards and adjust your focus at the posterior globe level. Retinal detachment will appear as a thin, straight, or wavy line displaced from the inner surface of the posterior globe. In this position, you can also see the optic nerve extending posteriorly and away from the globe. In the appropriate clinical context you can measure the optic nerve sheath diameter to assess for raised intracranial pressure. To achieve this, measure the optic nerve sheath diameter 3mm below its insertion into the globe to avoid

where it flares into the base of the globe. An optic nerve sheath diameter at this level over 5mm is abnormal and is both sensitive and specific for raised intracranial pressure[2]. Sometimes a little air trapped beneath the eyelid will prevent visualization of the deeper structures. If the patient is able, get them to blink a couple of times to try and clear this. As with any paired structure, ultrasound examination of the asymptomatic, contralateral side might be valuable for comparison.

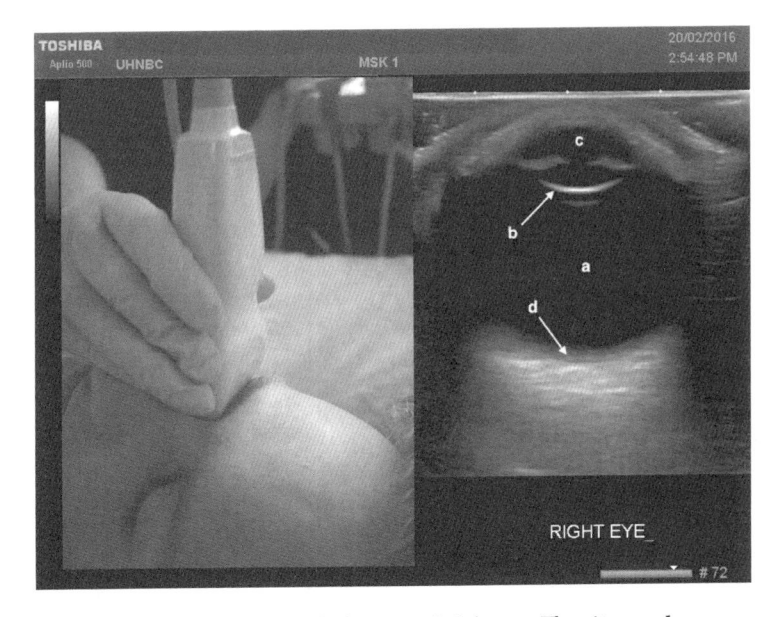

Figure 15. Ocular ultrasound of a normal right eye. The vitreous humour (a) of the eye is demonstrated as anechoic space. The echogenic, linear structure seen in the near field represents the lens (b) with the aqueous humour (c) anterior to it. Posteriorly lies the retina (d).

Chapter 10
Early Obstetrics (OB)

Probe:
Low-frequency curvilinear

Preset:
Early OB or OB 1st Trimester

Positioning:
Supine. Ask the patient to lower pants to below the pubic bone.

Prep:
A full bladder is essential to transabdominal early obstetrical ultrasound scan. Have the patient drink 1 litre of water to fill the bladder.

Technique:
As described in the pelvic ultrasound chapter, a full bladder is necessary for good visualization of early obstetrical structures.

Apply gel to the probe and place on patient's abdomen, just above the pubic bone, in the sagittal position. Provided that the patient's bladder is optimally full, you will see a dark structure that represents the fluid-filled bladder. Just posterior to the bladder you should see the uterus. Depending on the gestational age of the pregnancy, you might see a gestational sac in the fundus of the uterus, which contains a fetal pole with a yolk sac. Ultrasound is able to see a gestation transabdominally at approximately 6 weeks, or when serum β-HCG levels are approximately 1800 miU/ml or greater. For the purpose of simplicity, we will discuss OB scanning under 8 weeks gestational age and then at 12 weeks and over, as the scanning approaches differ depending on the gestational age of the embryo. To begin assessment of the uterus, position the probe sagittally on the patient. When you have identified the uterus, sweep from right to left to assess the whole uterus and locate the gestational sac. Turn the probe 90° to the transverse position and sweep low from the bladder and up to fundus of the uterus. You should see the anechoic gestational sac in the fundus.

Maternal Adnexae

Location and assessment of the ovaries is included in early obstetrical scans, especially if there is clinical concern for an ectopic pregnancy. The easiest method for locating the ovaries is to turn the probe transverse and scan low from the patient's bladder, angling the camera up and oblique slightly to the side you are assessing. Ovaries are almond-like in shape, approximately 3-5 centimeters in length, and echogenic with multiple anechoic cysts representing the follicles. Once you have located what you believe is the ovary, carefully turn the probe into the sagittal plane, keeping the image centered on the ovary, and sweep through side to side. Ovaries can be difficult to locate, even for experienced technologists, and structures such as bowel or pelvic floor muscles can often be mistaken for ovaries.

OB Under 8 Weeks Gestational Age (GA)

At this early stage, the goal is to assess the location of the gestational sac and determine fetal viability. The gestational sac should appear as an anechoic structure in the fundus of the uterus. You might see a fetal pole within the gestational sac as a small oblong structure. Often a small, bright, ring-shaped yolk sac can be seen adjacent to the fetal pole. Although only limited anatomy might be seen, cardiac motion should be apparent. Look for a flickering motion and measure with M-mode to determine the fetal heart rate (FHR). Drop the cursor in line within the fetal heart. The M-mode image will display a linear correlation of the motion of the heart. To calculate the fetal heart rate, pick two repeating points on the tracing, place a digital calliper on one and then another calliper on the next, and this will calculate the FHR automatically. Be sure to use only M-mode to detect the fetal heart rate and not pulse wave (PW) Doppler. PW Doppler exposes the fetus to a higher amount of energy and while there are no proven harmful effects from the use of ultrasound, it is considered best practice to expose the fetus to as little energy as possible. This is especially important during the first trimester, as this is when organ development occurs. To calculate the gestational age of the embryo, use the calculation package on the machine and select crown-rump length (CRL). As expected by the name of this measurement, place your callipers at the "head" and "rump" of the fetal pole, ideally in a sagittal plane. When assessing the embryo, look for dark fluid around the gestational sac, as this might represent a sub-chorionic hemorrhage, which is a common cause for per-vaginal bleeding in the first trimester.

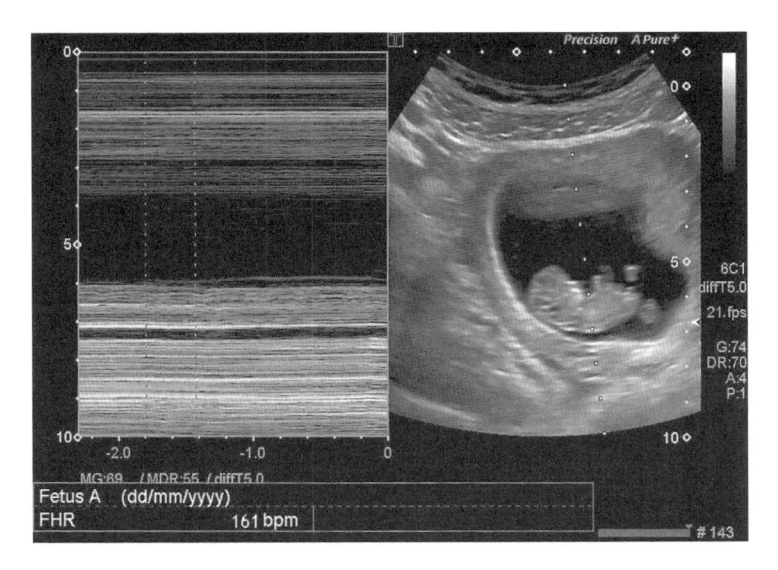

Figure 16. The above image demonstrates M-mode image of fetal heart rate on a 10-week gestational age embryo. The image on the right demonstrates a sagittal view of the embryo.

Tip

During assessment for an ectopic pregnancy, there are several ultrasound findings that might raise concern for an ectopic in a patient with the appropriate β-HCG levels and clinical presentation. Primarily, an empty uterus with no intrauterine gestation is seen accompanied by thickening of the endometrium, which represents the decidual reaction to the pregnancy. Additionally, a mass seen in the adnexa or adjacent to the ovary increases the likelihood of ectopic pregnancy. Finally, the presence of large volume of dark free fluid in the pelvis again raises suspicion. Beginners can find diagnosis of an ectopic pregnancy difficult and you should always consider obtaining confirmation with a formal ultrasound scan.

OB Over 12 Weeks GA

At approximately 12 weeks gestational age, the fetus has grown too large to be measured accurately by the CRL. You can now measure the gestational age of the fetus using four parameters: the head circumference, biparietal diameter, abdominal circumference and femur length. These measurements are more complex to perform, and perhaps outside the scope of this book. At this stage in fetal development, you can see more anatomical detail such as limbs, stomach, bladder, and fetal heart. The placenta will have developed, taking over the task of providing nutrition for the fetus. Placental tissue is typically bright on ultrasound and is attached to the uterine wall. The placenta can implant in any position in the uterus, anteriorly, posteriorly, or laterally. You should obtain a follow-up study if the placenta appears to be previa; that is implanted low near the cervix or completely covering the cervical os. Placenta previa can be a source of bleeding per vagina (PV). Amniotic fluid appears dark on ultrasound and there should be a generous amount visible around the fetus.

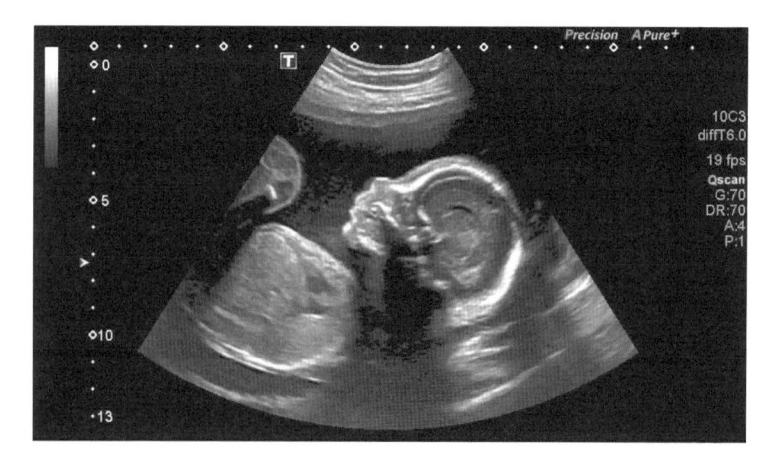

Figure 17. Sagittal image of a 20-week gestational age fetus. The fetal facial profile is demonstrated.

Tip

If you intend to measure the fetus to determine gestational age, don't forget to input the patients last menstrual period (LMP) or the estimated date of delivery (EDD) into the ultrasound unit. Most units have an input option at the home screen when the patient is selected from the work list. By entering the LMP, the unit calculates the approximate gestational age giving a basis for comparison for any measurements obtained. It should be noted that once the patient has had a dating ultrasound in the first trimester, it is best practice use the calculated due date from this scan as a reference for future ultrasonic fetal growth measurements as it is considered more accurate than using the LMP.

Chapter 11
Late Obstetrics (OB)

Probe:
Low-frequency curvilinear

Preset:
OB General or OB 2/3rd Trimester

Positioning:
Supine. Ask the patient to lower pants to hips and below the pubic bone. This will allow better visualization of the cervix, provided the patient's bladder is sufficiently full.

Prep:
A full bladder will aid visualization of the cervix. Ask the patient to drink approximately 1 litre of water to fill the bladder.

Technique:

Apply gel to the probe and place sagittally on patient's abdomen, just above the pubic bone. If the patient's bladder is full, you will see a dark structure representing the bladder with the endocervical canal deep to it. It is important to assess the cervix to ensure it is long and closed. Greater than 3 centimeters is considered the normal value for cervical length. Any less than this raises concern for cervical incompetence and pre-term labour. If the cervix is shortening, you might see dark fluid in the upper endocervical canal, creating a beaking or funnelling effect. This is cause for concern and warrants further investigation.

You can also determine the fetal position at this time, as you will either see the fetal head by the cervix; cephalic position, or you will see the lower extremities; breech position. Now move the probe upwards toward the maternal umbilicus to determine the placental location. The placenta can be in any position, posterior, anterior, or lateral. It is important to make sure the placenta edge is not near the cervix, as placenta previa puts the patient at high risk for hemorrhage during delivery. During placental visualization, you can assess for abruption. Placenta abruption occurs when the placenta separates from the uterine wall. This can be very subtle on ultrasound and is challenging for even experienced scanners. The normal placenta has a hypoechoic layer between the placenta and the uterus and this is known as the retro-placental complex. When abruption occurs, there is a loss of the retro-placental complex and there is often a dark, fluid collection present between the placenta and the uterine wall.

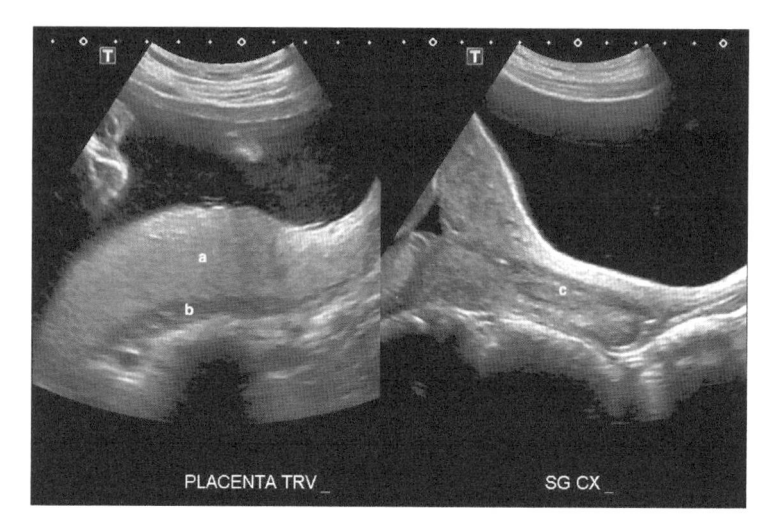

Figure 18. The dual-screen image above shows the normal cervix and placenta. On the left, the placental (a) is positioned posteriorly and a hypoechoic layer representing the retro-placental complex (b) is seen between the placenta and the uterine wall. On the right image, a long and closed cervix (c) is seen.

Now it is time to assess the fetus. The fetus is much more developed compared to early obstetrical scans, and you can only see small portions of the fetus at a time. Obstetrical scanning presents a unique challenge different from ultrasound of the abdomen or pelvis, because the target of the ultrasound does not lie in traditional scanning planes. The fetus can lie in any position within the uterus, and is also mobile. A good place to start is with the fetal head. Find the fetal head, and line it up sagittally on the fetus so you can see the skull and the cervical spine. To assess the fetal heart rate, move the probe caudally on the fetus. As you scan into the fetal thorax you will see a moving, anechoic structure; this is the fetal heart. Again, apply M-mode to measure the fetal heart rate.

You can assess the volume of amniotic fluid subjectively by looking for at least one generous pocket of fluid. However, if the fluid volume appears low, a measurement of the Single Deepest Pocket (SDP) can provide a quantitative measure. When measuring the amniotic fluid, it is important to keep the probe at 90° to the patient for an accurate measurement. Select the largest pocket of dark fluid and measure it anterior to posterior. Make sure not to include any limbs or umbilical cord within the pocket of fluid. A SDP of less than 2 centimeters is considered oligohydramnios and further assessment is needed to determine fetal well-being. If you see no fluid surrounding the fetus (anhydramnios,) this is cause for concern indicating potential premature rupture of membranes (PROM) and preterm labour. Findings of anhydramnios might require an emergency caesarean section.

Signs of Fetal Well-being

When performing an obstetrical ultrasound, there are several indicators that are reassuring for fetal well being. Primarily, of course, is the presence of a strong fetal heart rate at approximately 120-180 beats per minute (bpm). Secondary signs include fetal movement, such as rolls, turns, kicks etc., fetal tone, i.e. opening and closing of hands, and fetal breathing, as seen by contraction of the diaphragm and the belly moving in and out.

Chapter 12
Cardiac Sonography

Probe:
Phased

Preset:
Echo or Cardiac

Positioning:
Left lateral decubitus initially, then supine. Attach 3 lead ECG to patient for cardiac rhythm.

Technique:
Cardiac sonography or echocardiography is a specialized ultrasound examination of the heart. Depending on local expertise, echocardiography (or echo for short) is usually interpreted by cardiologists, internists, or radiologists. The method of the examination differs from general sonography in that instead of storing predominantly static images, you acquire cine-loops of a single beat from the cardiac cycle. The full echo examination is lengthy

and requires advanced technique, includes many complex measurements, and involves viewing the heart from multiple angles. The learning curve for echocardiography is hampered by often challenging visualization of structures in the average patient population. However, for the purposes of this book, we will describe the basic scanning planes, focusing on the applications of these views for assessment of right and left ventricular function, right atrial pressure quantification and pericardial effusions.

Echocardiography is the one case where you are allowed to break with convention and scan left-handed. Many echocardiographers are trained to scan left-handed. Primarily, ergonomics plays a large role in which hand is used to scan. When scanning left-handed, place the ultrasound unit on the left-hand side of the stretcher and roll the patient into the left-lateral decubitus position. When scanning left-handed, the patient faces you as you place the probe on his or her chest. Echo can be performed with your right hand and in this case, you would position the ultrasound unit on the right side of the patient and then reach over to the patient's left side. At times, right-handed scanning can place additional strain on your back and shoulder but the ability to scan with your dominant hand might be a greater advantage, especially for a beginner. With left-handed scanning, you are closer and have greater access to the structures of interest, but the required probe positioning might place strain on your wrist if not properly supported. The important thing is to be aware of the ergonomics when performing echo and pick the position that is most comfortable for you.

Patient positioning is very important in an echocardiogram. It can be very challenging to obtain the proper views when scanning patients solely in the supine position. Begin with the patient supine and attach a three-lead ECG to provide the cardiac rhythm. This will allow you to image and monitor the entire cardiac cycle. Then roll the patient into a left lateral decubitus position, with his or her left arm tucked under his or her head to provide access to the chest.

Parasternal

There are three main scanning positions for an echocardiography scan, the parasternal window, the apical window and the subcostal window. The parasternal window is located just left of the sternum in between the ribs at approximately the 3rd or 4th intercostal space. You can hold the probe in either long axis or short axis, depending on the position of the indicator notch on the probe. By turning the probe so that the indicator is pointing towards the patient's right shoulder, you will obtain the parasternal long axis (PLAX) view. By scanning between the ribs in the PLAX window, you will be able to see an oblique view of the heart focusing on the left heart.

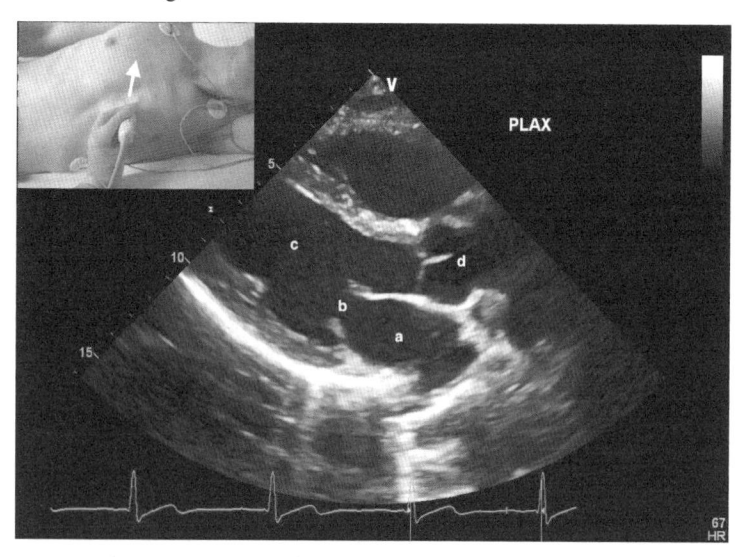

Figure 19. Parasternal long axis of the heart. As shown in the insert image in the left hand corner, the probe indicator is pointing towards the patient's right shoulder (see arrow). The PLAX view demonstrates the structures of the left heart including the left atrium (a), mitral valve (b), left ventricle (c), and the aortic valve (d).

You can assess the left ventricle (LV) in the short axis plane by turning the probe and indicator 90°. You can now see all walls of the left ventricle in cross-sectional slices, known as parasternal short axis (PSAX) view. By sweeping up towards the patient's head, you will be able to assess the aortic valve in transverse, the tricuspid valve and the pulmonary valve. By sweeping towards the patient's feet, you can visualize the mitral valve and the left ventricle from the basal to the apical level.

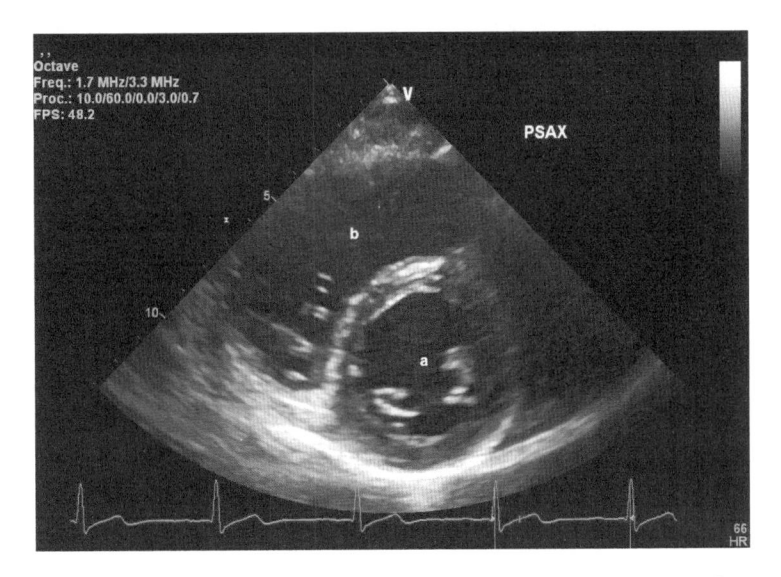

Figure 20. Parasternal short axis view at the level of the papillary muscles. Left ventricle is seen in short axis (a) with all walls visible. The right ventricle (b) is also seen.

Apical

The second window utilized in echocardiography is the apical window. This window is best located by finding the apical pulse, typically near the 5th intercostal space. Place the probe laterally on the patient's ribs, using the palpable apical pulse as a guide. The indicator should be pointing straight down, towards the floor. In the apical four-chamber view (4CH), the apex of the heart is at the top of the screen and the atria at the bottom of the screen.

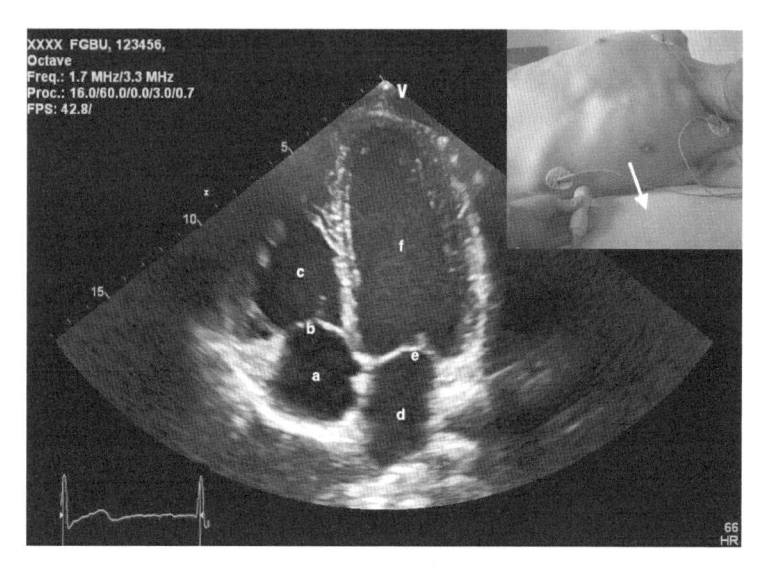

Figure 21. Apical 4CH view. The probe is now positioned laterally on the patient, with the indictor pointing downwards (see insert arrow). Right and left heart structures are demonstrated. Shown are the right atrium (a), the tricuspid valve (b), and the right ventricle (c), left atrium (d), mitral valve (e), and left ventricle (f).

You can obtain several other views using the apical window by rotating the indicator in increments of 90°. This allows you to see other cross-sectional planes of the left heart. For example, by turning the probe 90° counter-clockwise, the image will reflect the left heart in an apical two-chamber view (2CH). By further turning the probe another 90° counter-clockwise the image will demonstrate the apical three-chamber view (3CH) and essentially providing views of the same structures as a PLAX view. Apical 2CH and 3CH are advanced techniques and for the purpose of simplicity, will not be discussed further.

Subcostal

Finally, the last cardiac scanning plane discussed here is the subcostal view. For this view, with the patient in a supine position, place the probe just inferior to the xiphoid process of the sternum with the indicator pointing to the patient's left. If you apply gentle pressure and scan up towards the patient's head and under the sternum, you will obtain the subcostal four-chamber view. The subcostal window is by far the easiest window to achieve without rib shadows to work around. A large, held inspiration by the patient greatly improves the visibility through this window.

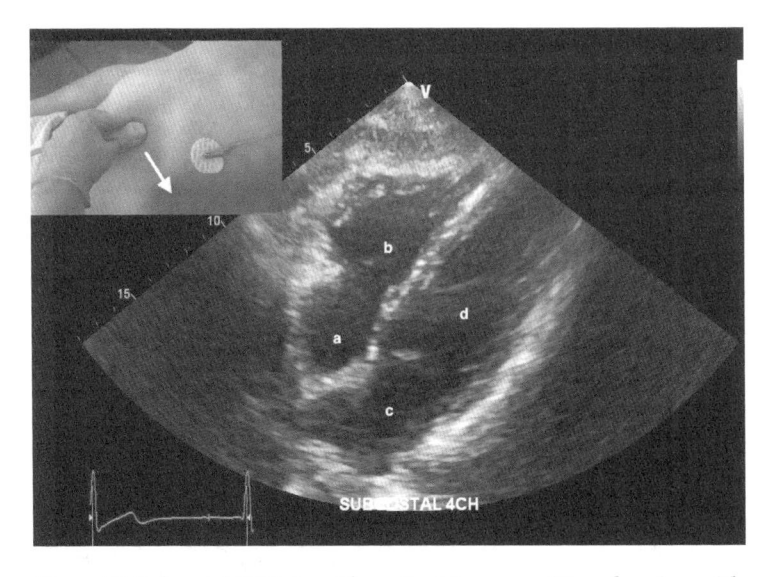

Figure 22. Subcostal 4CH view. The patient is now positioned supine, with the probe placed subcostally and indicator pointing to patient's left (see insert arrow). The subcostal view demonstrates a 4CH view similar to the Apical 4CH. In the right heart, the right atrium (a) and ventricle (b) are shown. In the left heart, the left atrium (c) and ventricle (d) are shown.

Right Heart Ventricular Function

From the apical 4CH view, you can assess and quantify right ventricular function. Using M-mode, you can drop a cursor through the free wall of the RV at the level of the tricuspid annulus. The corresponding M-mode image shows the up and down motion of the right ventricle (RV), and by placing callipers on the peak and the base of the image, you can determine the excursion of the wall. This measurement is known as TAPSE (Tricuspid Annular Plane Systolic Excursion), and a normal value is greater than 16 mm[3]. If the TAPSE is low *and* this corresponds with visual assessment, this is indicative of right ventricular systolic dysfunction.

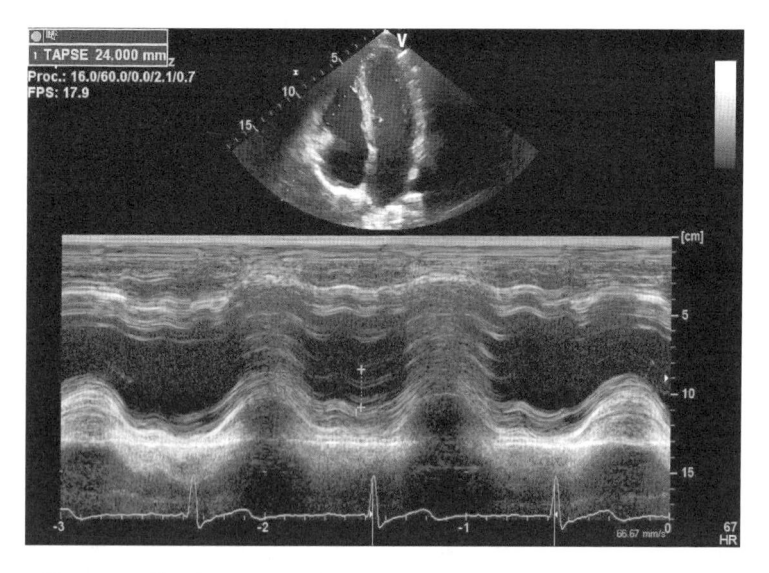

Figure 23. The above image shows a normal TAPSE of 24 mm. M-mode measurement of the right ventricular function has been performed by placing the cursor through the RV wall.

Left Ventricular Function

In order to assess left ventricular function, you should visualize all walls of the LV. This can be difficult to accomplish for beginners. You can calculate the LV ejection fraction (normal is greater than 55%) formally using the Simpsons Biplane method for determining LV function[4]. This measurement however, is dependent on very good visualization of the LV walls in apical 4CH and 2CH. Furthermore, the calculation is heavily user dependent and can be inconsistent. Instead, we recommend beginners use a qualitative assessment of LV systolic function, assessing the parasternal SAX view at the level of the papillary muscles to see all the walls of the LV, and an apical 4CH view focusing on the LV. When assessing the movement of the endocardium visually, all segments of the wall should be contracting in systole and relaxing in diastole.

Tip

Either using a pencil or your finger, point to the center of the LV chamber on the PSAX ventricle view. Are all the segments contracting inward towards the point? If so, function is likely normal.

For more advanced users, there is an additional qualitative assessment of the ejection fraction available. Begin by obtaining an apical 4CH view. Divide the LV into six segments, representing the basal, mid, and apical walls of the inter-ventricular septum and posterior lateral wall of the LV respectively. By individually assessing the wall motion of each segment and designating it a numerical value, the sum of this value can determine a rough estimate of the ejection fraction. For example, if the wall segment is contracting normally, assign it a value of 10. If it is hypokinetic assign a value of 5, if akinetic, assign a value of

0. In a heart with normal systolic function, each segment will be assigned a value of 10, which when totalled will equal 60, thus corresponding to a normal ejection fraction of 60%. This process is repeated in the apical 2CH view to assess the anterior and inferior walls of the LV. By performing this technique in 4CH and 2CH, you can assess all wall segments for regional wall motion abnormalities. An average of the two totals provides an estimate of global LV ejection fraction.

Tip

To get the best visualization of the LV in apical 4CH, decrease the depth centering on just the LV and move the focus towards the apex. Held inspiration or expiration can help reduce lung artefact.

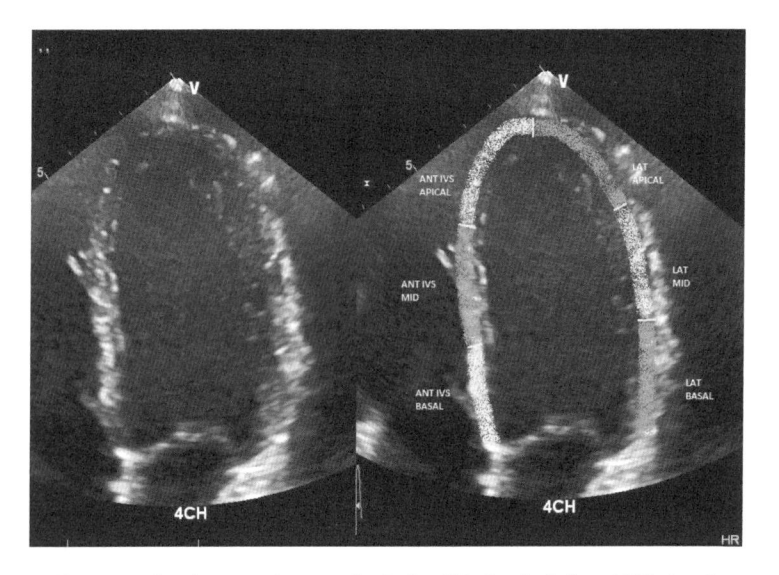

Figure 24. Dual-screen image of apical 4CH. On the left, a 4CH view is shown, focusing on the LV. On the right, the six different LV wall segments are annotated.

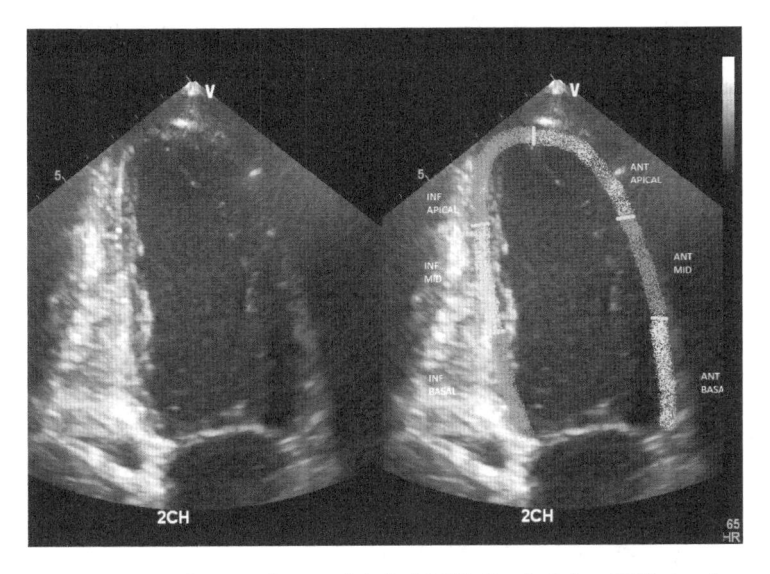

Figure 25. Dual-screen image of Apical 2CH. On the left, a 2CH view is show, focusing on the LV. On the right, again the six different segments of the LV wall are annotated. By assessing the LV walls in 4CH and 2CH, as described above, an estimation of ejection fraction can be calculated.

Right Atrial Pressure (RAP)

From the subcostal window, you can visualize the inferior vena cava (IVC). By turning the probe 90° to the right so that the indicator is pointing up towards the patient's head, you can see the proximal portion of the IVC, as well as the right atrium and left lobe of the liver. You can perform an indirect assessment of the RAP by looking for collapse of the IVC during inspiration and at the size of the IVC. A normal RAP of 3 mmHg is represented by an IVC measuring less than 21 mm in AP dimension and which collapses more than 50% during a quick inspiration, or "sniff". If the IVC is dilated, but still collapses more than 50%, the RAP can be estimated at 8 mmHg. However, if the IVC is dilated and does not collapse, this indicates elevated right heart pressure, and the RAP can be estimated at 15 mmHg[3].

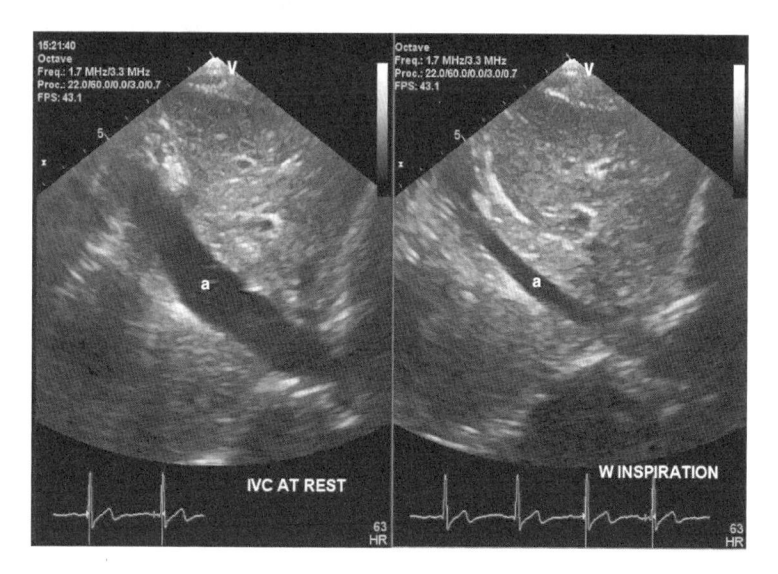

Figure 26. Dual-screen image of IVC at rest and with inspiration. As shown above, the IVC (a) collapses with inspiration and is not dilated, therefore demonstrating a normal right atrial pressure (RAP).

Pericardial Effusion

Assessment for pericardial effusion is certainly one of the most useful common applications of the subcostal window through which you can see the pericardial space (and fluid if present) both anteriorly and posteriorly. When there is a significant pericardial effusion greater than 2 cm in depth, look for anechoic fluid around the myocardium of the heart. Significant pericardial effusions can cause tamponade and restrict the filling of the right heart. If a large pericardial effusion is present and tamponade is suspected, look for collapse of the right heart during systole and even paradoxical movement of the inter-ventricular septum (IVS) towards the left ventricle.

Chapter 13
Ultrasound-Guided Procedures

One of the largest growth areas in the use of diagnostic ultrasound over recent years has been as a tool for performing invasive and interventional procedures more safely and accurately. The portable nature of ultrasound units combined with the ability to see the relative position of both the target and the advancing needle in real time, gives ultrasound operators an advantage over other forms of image guidance such as MRI and CT. In this chapter we will provide some useful techniques for guiding needles with ultrasound starting with simple methods and increasing in complexity as the operator's skill level rises to match. This chapter will not cover important patient pre-procedural and safety steps such as obtaining informed consent, checking patient medications, and assessing complication risk such as bleeding or infection. Nor will it cover important procedural steps such as prepping the skin and maintaining a sterile field, as it is assumed that the readers will already be familiar with this. When learning interventional techniques such as these outlined below, performing procedures under the direct supervision of an experienced trainer is always advisable until you have gained appropriate experience. This chapter provides only guidance and should not be considered as a substitute for directly supervised training.

Scan and Mark

This is the easiest technique to master and one that even the most accomplished interventionalists use when the conditions are appropriate. When the target is large, such as a large simple pleural effusion or extensive free ascites, you can use the low-frequency curvilinear probe to scan for the deepest, largest pocket of fluid a safe distance from surrounding vital structures. You should allow some safety margin for the patients breathing which might cause some movement of the target collection. Once located, freeze the image and measure the depth from skin to the edge of the target using on-screen callipers. Mark a cross or dimple on the skin directly under the probe and over the target area, then put the ultrasound probe away. Prepare and anesthetize the skin. Advance the needle or catheter into the patient from the marked spot on the skin down to the required depth until you can aspirate the target fluid through the needle. It is best to advance the needle a few millimeters more than the measured target depth to account for some skin thickening secondary to the local anesthetic and some puckering of the chest or abdominal wall soft tissues ahead of the needle tip before it penetrates the fluid pocket. Once the needle tip is in the fluid pocket, you can aspirate a diagnostic sample or if preferred, insert a guide-wire, dilate up a track to appropriate size, and insert a drainage catheter using Seldinger technique[5] if desired.

This technique works well when draining large fluid collections or placing suprapubic catheters in severely dilated bladders and can be modified for liver biopsies for acute and chronic (but not focal) liver disease. The advantages of this technique are that it is quick and does not require the use of a sterile probe cover. The main disadvantage is that the target collection must be reasonably large, as you do not guide the needle under direct visualization.

In terms of patient positioning, with needle aspiration of pleural fluid, try sitting the patient up at the far edge of the bed with their legs over the side and have them lean over a pillow on a table. This allows you room to scan and perform the aspiration from a posterior approach. If the patient is unable to sit up, try rolling them onto his or her left side or using a lateral approach if the effusion is large.

With needle aspiration of intra-abdominal ascites, lay the patient supine and access the fluid in the left or right lower quadrants of the abdomen. Two centimeters superior and medial to the anterior superior iliac spine of the pelvis is a good starting point and avoids most vital structures. You should pick the largest pocket of fluid as possible for needling. Try tipping the bed slightly head up using gravity to drain the fluid down into the lower abdomen and pelvis and increase the size of the fluid pocket. You can also roll the patient onto one side or the other to increase the pooling effect further.

Tip

After scanning for the best place to anesthetize and insert the needle, mark the skin by applying pressure with the end of a plastic straw directly onto the skin. This leaves a temporary, circular dimple on the skin, which lasts long enough for you to start your invasive procedure and doesn't wash off with skin prep solutions unlike marks made with pen and ink. The plastic, protective, tubular sheaths that come with needle/catheter sets or procedure kits (and which are usually discarded) are great for this.

Cross-plane needle guidance

This technique represents a step up in complexity and is more suited to smaller and more superficial targets in the body such as venous or arterial catheterization. This technique does allow for real-time visualization of the advancing needle tip and visual confirmation as it enters the target vessel.

The best probe to use here is a linear, high or medium-frequency probe, which is placed over and across the target vessel at a 90° angle to the long axis of the vessel. Use a vascular or superficial small parts preset and position the focus at the level of the target. The target vessel will appear as a round or oval structure directly beneath the probe. Identify the target vessel. Veins collapse under mild pressure. Arteries do not compress easily and visually pulsate. If in doubt, apply color Doppler to be sure. It is important to orientate the probe correctly according to the image on the screen so that small movements of the probe in one direction result in corresponding movements of the image in the appropriate direction. By using the same convention routinely, you will build up your hand-eye ultrasound coordination skills much more rapidly. Use a sterile probe cover. This serves two purposes. Firstly, it helps maintain a sterile field at the site of skin puncture, and secondly it protects the probe from contamination by body fluids.

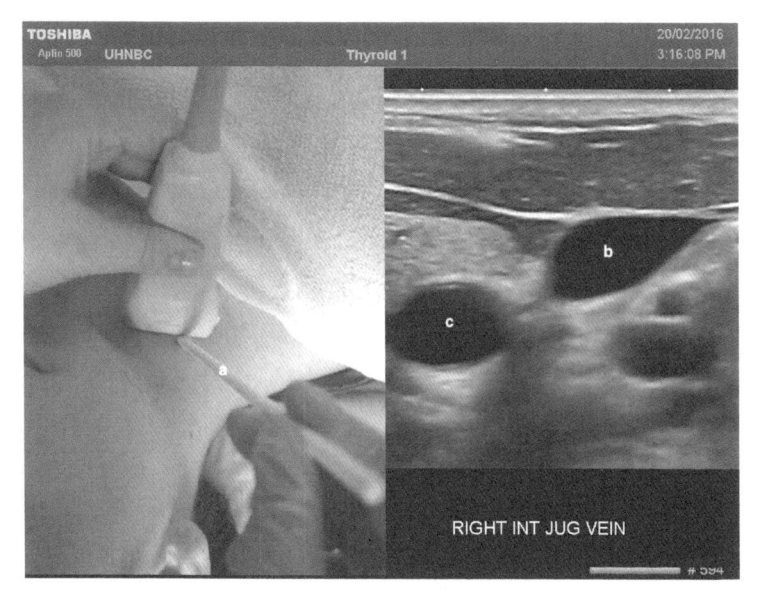

Figure 27. Short axis cross-plane needle guidance. Anatomical view from top of bed. Probe is placed transverse on patient's neck. Pointer (a) indicates the path of needle which is inserted at the side of the probe. On the ultrasound image, the internal jugular vein is seen as a teardrop-shaped, anechoic structure (b) adjacent to the more round-shaped common carotid artery (c).

Fitting a sterile probe cover

Sterile probe covers usually look like a long plastic sheath with a blind end. To fit a sterile probe cover, the easiest way is to find a second, non-sterile person to assist you. The goal is to get non-sterile gel on the probe tip, the probe cover over this and then sterile gel on the outside between the covered probe and patient's prepped skin. If air gets between the probe and cover, you will not be able to see an image on the screen during scanning.

After you have put on sterile gloves, pick up the probe cover from your sterile procedure tray. They usually come folded.

Bunch up and concertina the cover into a short donut shaped ring. Hold the cover by the blind end and then invert the bunched up cover inside out and back over the same hand and glove. Ask your assistant to place some non-sterile gel on the scanning surface of the probe and hold it up in front of you, with the gel pointing upwards. With your fingers at the blind end of the cover, grab the tip of the probe through the cover and then with your other hand grab the very edge of the free end of the cover. Next, pull down and unravel the bunched-up cover back off your hand and down over the probe and lead, straightening out the cover as you go. If you have one, use a sterile elastic band to hold the cover onto the probe tightly. Try and unravel the whole length of the cover when fitting. Otherwise, it is easy to double up the cover over the probe head and accidentally trap a thin layer of air between the two layers, which prevents an image forming when scanning.

Infiltrating local anesthetic

With the probe held tangential to the skin and transversely over the vessel or target, infiltrate your local anesthetic at a point half way down the side of the probe and over the vessel. Do this on the side of the probe, which gives you a clear view of the needle at the skin. Angle the needle slightly so that it's tip passes under the probe and through the scan plane. On the screen you should see the movement of the soft tissues as the needle passes through. The tip itself is often difficult to see as it lies at a steep angle to the scan plane. Visualization of the needle tip position can be accentuated by jiggling the needle back and forth a little, which causes movement of the soft tissues immediately around the needle tip. Infiltrate the local anesthetic superficial to the vessel. This will be visible as a dark, lens-shaped collection of fluid.

Main procedure

Once anesthetized, and with the probe in the same position, make a nick in the skin with a scalpel blade if required. Insert your puncture needle at the same location relative to the probe and vessel as for the anesthetic needle earlier, i.e. half way along the side of the probe and angling slightly under the probe. On the screen you should be able to see the position of the needle tip descend as you advance it by the motion of the surrounding tissues. If you lined up the mid point of the probe and vessel correctly, the needle should descend down onto and into the vessel lumen. The needle tip may buckle the front wall of the vessel necessitating a small, quick jab to fully enter the lumen. The needle tip should be more easily seen when it is the vessel lumen. If you are having trouble seeing the tip, gently rock the probe back and forth scanning up and down the needle until you see its tip. Jiggling the needle will again help localize its tip position.

When accessing veins, do not press down too hard with the probe or you will compress the vein making your target smaller and more difficult to hit. If your needle accidentally passes right through the vessel, pull back until the tip is in the lumen. With venous access, it is useful to have a syringe on the end of the needle. When the tip is in the venous lumen, you should be able to withdraw venous blood into the syringe easily. When accessing an artery, no syringe is required, as blood should start spurting from the empty needle hub in a pulsatile manner when the tip is intraluminal.

Common difficulties encountered with this method are firstly, difficulty lining up all three components, the needle, the mid-point of the probe, and the vessel at the mid-point of the screen image and secondly, visualizing the needle tip as it descends below the probe and intersects the thin scan plane. As with all these image-guided procedures, practice makes perfect.

Tip

A safe way to practice ultrasound-guided procedures is to use a hand-made practice phantom such as an olive or grape buried in a chicken breast fillet. This will allow you to develop the bilateral hand-eye coordination required to perform these safely before moving onto real patients.

In-plane needle guidance

This method requires the greatest degree of skill and practice to perform well. Instead of inserting the needle along the side of the probe, this technique sees the needle inserted at one end of the probe, and then guided entirely within the scan plane and visualized on screen all the way to the target. This technique is more suited to small or deeper targets where greater accuracy is required such as nerve blocks and biopsy procedures. You can also puncture vessels with this technique if preferred.

Again, use a sterile probe cover. Localize your target with an initial scan and determine an access path from the skin at the edge of the screen image down and across the image to the target. The end of the probe at which you puncture the skin is usually dependent on the hand with which you intend to hold the needle. If right-handed, approach from the right side of both the probe and screen image, and vice versa if you are left-handed.

There are two ways to proceed at this point. Some machine manufacturers have a physical, probe-specific, needle-guide device, which clips onto the side of the probe and carries a channel held at a fixed angle. This device holds and guides the puncture needle within the scan plane. They are either disposable or reusable (in which case they require sterilization before each use). The ultrasound machine has a "biopsy guide" setting, which activates a fixed, oblique, dotted line on the screen image extending down from the edge of the probe. When used in conjunction with the correct needle-guide device, the dotted line predicts the on-screen path of the needle into the tissues. The dots are usually calibrated at one-centimeter intervals making the distance-to-target and length of needle required easy to calculate. After instilling local anesthetic, position the covered probe on the skin so that the target lies along the biopsy-guide trajectory path. Then pass the puncture or biopsy needle down the guide channel into the skin. This should be visible on the screen following the dotted line down to the target. When at the required depth, perform your biopsy or alternate procedure.

The second way to proceed is to use a free-hand method. In this case, there is no guide device and you must plot the needle path and guide the needle by watching the screen and advancing the needle under free-hand control. The challenge is to keep the needle in the scan plane and judge the angle and predicted path of the needle through the tissues. This is considerably more difficult to achieve, particularly when working at depth, and therefore requires more practice and experience to master. If the needle tip is difficult to see on screen, try jiggling the needle, as the induced movement of the soft tissues immediately around the needle tip is more easily seen than the needle tip itself. Another way to improve visualization of the needle is to bring up your focal zone marker from the level of the target to the level of the needle shaft.

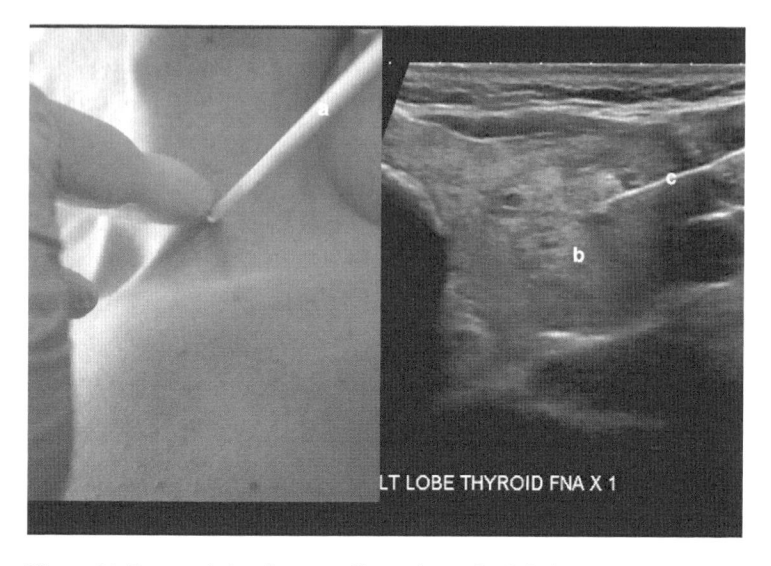

Figure 28. Long axis in-plane needle guidance for left thyroid gland biopsy procedure. The image is viewed from the patient's left, with probe placed transversely on the neck and pointer (a) representing the needle's path. On the right image, a left thyroid nodule (b) is shown in transverse with the biopsy needle (c).

Tip

When using the in-plane method of needle guidance, you will be able to see the needle more easily when the angle between the sound beam and the needle is closer to 90°, that is, at a shallow angle of approach. When the approach angle is steep and the needle pointed more vertically, the needle is more difficult to see. This is one reason why deeper targets are more difficult to hit. With deeper targets, it may be preferable to choose a longer needle and take a longer path-to-target if it allows you to use a more shallow approach angle. With curvilinear probes, you can also angle the probe at the skin to increase the beam-to-needle angle and improve needle visualization. Some newer machines have a "beam steering" function, which angulates the sound beam automatically, thus increasing the angle between the sound beam and the needle.

Safety point

When performing ultrasound-guided interventional procedures, extra time spent beforehand planning the procedure, the probe position, the puncture site, and the predicted needle path pays back dividends ten-fold later during the procedure. Measuring the depth of the target will inform your choice of needle length. You should look for any vital structures to be avoided in the vicinity, such as vessels, pleura, and solid organs before plotting your needle path accordingly to minimize the risk of inadvertent injury. Do not forget vital structures behind and deep to your target, particularly if you are using a biopsy needle which automatically extends or throws a central stylet a distance beyond an outer hollow needle.

Ultrasound guided drainage procedures

These deserve a special mention. We almost exclusively use what is known as Seldinger technique[5] for these procedures. With this technique a puncture needle is inserted with or without image guidance into the target fluid collection be it an abscess, seroma, empyema, pleural effusion, or dilated renal collecting system. Once in the correct position, a guide wire is inserted down the needle into the target collection to maintain access. The needle is then removed over the wire. Over the wire, a track is dilated through the tissues using dilators of increasing size before deploying a drainage catheter, again over the wire. After confirming position of the catheter with scanning, the wire is removed. The main advantage of Seldinger technique is that it is safer than using a catheter with a sharp, stiff trocar, which typically requires more force to insert. Also, once the wire is in position, access is assured and the process of dilating the track can be performed gently and gradually with less risk of injuring nearby structures.

When using ultrasound guidance to perform drainage catheter insertion, the same principles outlined previously, particularly with respect to insertion of the initial puncture needle, continue to apply. On initial assessment, you should identify the target dark appearing fluid collection and plot a safe needle path. If the collection contains gas, such as in the case of an abscess, the collection might be difficult to see due to the artefact generated by the gas. Changing the position of the patient or the angle of approach of the probe and needle might circumvent this, but often an alternative method of image guidance, such as CT will be more appropriate. If you are unable to see your target clearly with your initial scan, you should not attempt an ultrasound-guided approach.

Tip

When preparing for a drain insertion procedure, make sure you have all the required equipment **before** *you start. Check you have the syringes and needle for anesthetizing, a blade, puncture needle, guide wire, dilators, appropriate catheter for deployment, as well as a drainage bag and connecting tubes if required. Prepare your catheter beforehand, as it may need to be pre-straightened with a hollow central stiffener. Check you have the correct wire size that complements the other equipment. Do this by sliding everything over the wire and off again in turn making sure the other components run over the wire smoothly. Check the connectors are compatible. Do* *all this before you start, as there is nothing more frustrating than having to wait for a runner to go and fetch a vital, missing piece of kit while you have a needle or wire in a patient. Similarly, some pigtail catheters have a locking mechanism to prevent accidental displacement following insertion. If the catheter you are deploying is of the locking type, make sure you know how to operate this before you start the procedure and always document the catheter type in the patient's clinical record afterwards.*

Chapter 14
Choosing your new ultrasound machine

Choosing an ultrasound machine for purchase can feel like a complicated and daunting task. There are many current manufacturers of ultrasound equipment and when asked, each will gladly extol all the latest features on their machines and the advantages over their competitors. There is no doubt that the quality of images generated by every new generation of machine exceeds its predecessor. In addition, new features become available with each generation. Here, there are parallels to be drawn with purchasing a new car and a similar approach is required to help narrow down your choices. Like new cars, ultrasound machines are marketed to key user segments to meet their particular market needs. The key segments are generally as follows:

1. High-end "do it all and do it well" machines (hospital radiology departments)
2. Mid-range "do it all but on a budget" machines +/- portability (outpatient ultrasound clinics, ER rooms)
3. Low-end user-friendly machines (interventional room, emergency departments, ICU etc.)
4. Low-end hand-held machines (personal use, pocket sized)
5. Specialist machines

This stratification is an oversimplification and there are machines that undoubtedly cross over segments but it is a useful start. Generally speaking, when it comes to cost, you pay a premium for a greater number of features, higher image quality and greater portability. At the current time of writing, there is also a trade-off between the degree of portability and the number of features and image quality, although manufacturers are working hard to reduce this trade-off.

Before purchasing a machine you need to ask yourself the following questions: For what types of scans will I use the machine? For what pathologies will I be looking? How many different probes will I need? How important is portability to me? Are there any specific must-have features required for certain examinations I intend to perform?

Choosing the right probes is also an important consideration. To begin, we recommend purchasing a low-frequency curvilinear probe for general abdominal and pelvic work and a high-frequency linear probe for venous cannulation, MSK, testes, other small parts, and foreign-body work. A medium-frequency linear or "vascular" probe will be a useful addition for leg veins. If you intend to do cardiac work, we recommend the addition of a small footprint, cardiac phased-array probe. Beyond this, you are into the realm of more specialist probes such as endoluminal probes for transvaginal or endorectal imaging, hockey stick probes for superficial MSK, and neonatal probes for pediatrics. The extensive list of available probes can read like a long shopping list and it can be tempting to overspend on probes many of which might see only occasional use. Unless you do a lot of pelvic or pediatric work, the basic set of the first four probes mentioned above will cover 95% of your general scanning needs, especially if you are willing to be flexible and understand the controls on your machine well enough.

Once you have defined your requirements you can narrow down the required features such as:

- Multiple probe ports
- Color and power Doppler
- M-Mode
- Pulse wave Doppler
- Simple user interface
- Battery power
- Size, weight and portability
- Biopsy guide
- Data analytics e.g. fetal biometry and quantitative flow measurements
- Connectivity to networks and image storage and transfer
- Cost/Budget
- Different types of available probe

High-end machines

These are the workhorses of hospital radiology departments or busy clinics. They can do the full gamut of general studies ranging from vascular through musculoskeletal to obstetrical as well as interventional. They can be used with a vast array of different probes with specialist applications such as endoluminal imaging. They can be used for research and have the highest level of image quality and the greatest number of features. They usually require a high level of training to use effectively. They are also the most expensive and least portable machines. These are the flagship models of the manufacturers.

Mid-range machines

These can do most of the things that the high-end machines can do but have slightly fewer features and slightly lower image quality. They too can accept many different probes. Some manufacturers will allow the probes on their high-end and mid-range machines to be interchangeable. These are more suited to general outpatient clinics where the range of studies performed is relatively narrow but volume is high. These machines may also be the preferred option in Emergency Rooms and Obstetrical units where the users have already achieved at a high level of ultrasound proficiency. The cost of these machines is significantly lower than the high-end machines. Many manufacturers produce a portable "laptop" sized version of this level of machine, which is more suited to a mobile service and for technologists who must travel between sites. These laptop machines are also designed to dock with dedicated carts, which provide a stable base as well as extra probe ports and gel bottle holders.

Low-end user-friendly machines

These are typically found outside the ultrasound departments of hospitals and clinics. In the emergency room the need for data analytics or network connectivity can be sacrificed, replaced instead by a need for portability and a smaller footprint to allow positioning at the bedside. With fewer features to control, the manufacturers have concentrated on making these machines easy to use with fewer buttons and touch screen controls. They may still accept multiple probes, allowing a number of different scan types to be performed. Image quality varies but is generally lower than or similar to the mid-range machines. These machines are also commonly found in ICUs and interventional rooms for ultrasound-guided procedures. Their strength is in being able to provide exactly the required level of functionality to meet the specific needs of their users and no more, and being able to do this at a budget price point.

Low-end hand-held machines

This is a rapidly developing and exciting segment. Technological improvements have shrunk the size of the probes, and operating software can now be installed on small-screen devices the size of a cellphone or tablet. This truly brings ultrasound technology to a new level of accessibility. The number of features and image quality remains limited but is increasing with every generation. As processing power and data storage capacity improve according to Moore's Law, it is only a matter of time before these portable, pocket-sized machines will have similar capability to the current mid-range machines. These machines are the most likely candidates to replace the stethoscope in the pockets of the medical professionals of the future. For the time being however, these machines are best suited to those physicians who value portability above all other features and who perform a relatively narrow subset of bedside scan types. The price for these machines is the lowest of all but remains significant, perhaps out of reach of the casual user. This has led to some manufacturers offering lease or subscription-based contracts on these units, thus bringing the costs within reach of individual physicians.

Specialist Machines

These cater to niche applications such as superficial vascular access, endoscopic ultrasound, transesophageal echo or intravascular ultrasound. They are often optimized and limited to these functions and by definition less appropriate for general diagnostic use.

The Demonstration

Once you have defined your segment and listed the required features, the next step is to contact the manufacturers and arrange a demonstration. They will usually bring a demo unit to you, show you all the features, and let you try it on a few live cases. The importance of this step cannot be overemphasized as it provides you with an opportunity to assess the image quality, functionality, controls, and user-friendliness of the unit. It also provides the opportunity to ask questions about the included features and options. Some like to shortlist a few different units and manufacturers and try out several machines. Others may find a machine that suits their needs straightaway and move on to purchase. If you are unsure about certain features and your need for them, there is no harm in obtaining some advice from someone who has been through the evaluation and purchase process before, such as a peer, a colleague, or perhaps someone from your local radiology department.

Finally, consider important additional issues such as training, warranty, service, and maintenance. Who will perform this? Can maintenance be shared with local biomedical technicians? Does the manufacturer have service agents nearby? Do they provide rapid-access technical support and on-site training on how to use the unit? What would happen if the unit broke down or if a probe was dropped and damaged?

You should consider many things during the purchasing process but the key factor is user acceptance. The best machine is always one that you will actually enjoy using. There is no utility in having an expensive, highly specified machine if it never sees use and sits gathering dust in the corner of the department because no one can remember how to operate its controls.

Applications training and post purchase support

Receiving applications training soon after your new unit is delivered is crucial for learning how to use the machine effectively.

An applications specialist can do far more than just show you the controls. They can set up specific presets to suit your style of scanning, change default settings such cine clip recording to your preference, and upload reference databases for fetal biometry and obstetrical imaging. They can set up shortcuts or custom annotations to save you time. They will also give you tips on boot up, preset menus, battery life, and cleaning the machine and probes. Being present when your new machine is delivered for applications training should be made a priority. Learning to use the machine by reading the manufacturer's manual or second hand from another operator is never as effective.

Chapter 15
Troubleshooting and FAQs

This section is designed to act as a quick reference guide to help the reader when the machine doesn't seem to be working as it should. It takes the form of a checklist for the operator to run through when confronted with commonly encountered problems.

Nothing happens when I turn on the machine
- Check the machine is plugged into the electricity wall socket.
- If using a battery unit, recharge or replace the battery.
- Check you are pressing the correct button for on/off power.
- Call the biomedical engineering department to check the fuses.

I have plugged it in and turned it on. The warm up cycle has completed. The keyboard and dashboard lights are on but there is no image on the screen
- Check that the probe is plugged in correctly into the connector port.
- Some machines have more than one port and one is often set as the default port. Check there is a probe in this port.

I have an image but this does not move when I run my finger over the transducer surface
- Run your finger over any other probes connected to the machine to see if one of the other probes is currently selected.
- Check you have selected the correct probe on the dashboard.
- Check the freeze button isn't on (this is a common problem).
- If you have fitted a sterile probe cover, check that there is good contact with gel both between the probe and the inside of the cover and on the outside between the cover and skin.
- If you have fitted a sterile probe cover, check that you have not "doubled up" the cover on the probe accidentally placing two layers of the plastic cover over the transducer surface separated by a thin layer of air.

I have a moving image now but the image quality is very poor
- Apply more contact gel.
- Apply a little more pressure with the probe while respecting the patient's comfort.
- Check that you have the correct preset selected for the specific body part you are imaging.
- Check you have the depth set correctly for the body part and tissue you are interested in seeing.
- Make sure you have adjusted the focus to the correct depth
- Press the image optimization button if you have one or increase the gain
- If you are scanning an abdomen, move away from the midline where you may be encountering bowel gas or free

intraperitoneal air. Elsewhere check you are not scanning immediately over a bony structure.
- If the deeper structures appear too dark, change to a lower frequency on the same probe or switch to a different probe with a lower frequency.
- If not automatically on, turn on the harmonic or compound imaging functions.

I have a moving image but the image has a time lag and is "jerky"
- Check you are using the correct preset for the appropriate body part. For example, scanning an abdomen on a vascular preset will result in a "laggy" or "jerky" image.
- Check you have not accidentally turned on the Doppler. Adding color or pulse wave Doppler to a B-mode image (Duplex or Triplex imaging) automatically results in a reduction in the frame rate and a "jerky" image, because the machine has to perform more functions at the same time with the sound beam.

Why can't I save or print a frozen image?
- Some machines will not allow an image to be saved or printed if a patient's name has not been entered into the demographics screen and an appropriate image file/folder has not been generated.
- Check the printer is turned on, is connected and has paper.

Why can't I generate and save a cine clip?
- Some machines are set to capture cine clips prospectively, where you push the cine record button, scan the area, then repress the same button or freeze to end the clip. Other machines capture cine retrospectively, where pushing the cine button will automatically save the last 30 seconds of

scanning before you pushed the button. The length of the saved clip in this case is set as a default or set up when you originally bought the machine and can be varied.

When I am scanning, I get black lines or long shadows coming down vertically from the transducer surface over the length of the image

- Apply more gel to the skin surface to improve contact.
- If the shadows are at the edge of the screen, this part of the probe may have poor contact with the skin. Press down more firmly or rock the probe a little to improve contact or apply more gel here.
- If you are using a sterile probe cover, apply more gel to the transducer surface beneath the probe cover.
- Check you are not scanning over a bony structure such as a rib.
- If the black line is very thin and stays in the same place wherever you are scanning, this is likely to represent a broken crystal in the transducer array. This often occurs after someone accidentally drops the probe. You will either have to live with this or replace the probe.

I can find the area of interest but I can only see part of it, the rest seems obscured

This is where an ultrasound operator earns their stripes. The most common reasons for this are suboptimal positioning of the probe or patient and either intervening air in the lungs, bowel gas, or bony structures.

- Try changing the position or angle of the probe away from the lungs, bowel, or bony structures.
- Ask the patient to take a deep breath in or out to reveal more of the target structures.
- Change the position of the patient, either tilting up one side of the chest or moving them onto their side.

- Apply sustained gentle pressure with the probe to displace air in bowel away from your probe.

Other general tips
- Turn, sit, or stand patients up and use gravity to help you assess for fluid in the chest or abdomen and when assessing for inguinal hernias or leg veins.
- Ask the patient to perform a Valsalva manoeuvre when assessing for hernias or varicocele.
- Don't be afraid to change to a lower-frequency probe if you need more depth. Switch to a higher-frequency probe if you need to see more detail with superficial structures.
- When scanning musculoskeletal structures, move the appropriate digit, joint, or tendon to help localize pathology and confirm the anatomy while scanning in real time.
- With paired structures, scanning the contralateral, non-symptomatic side can be useful for comparison.
- Use the dynamic nature of real-time ultrasound to the full. You will see the movement of veins compressing under probe pressure more easily than the contents of the veins themselves.
- When in doubt, apply color or power Doppler. It will help solve a diagnostic problem more often than you think.
- Everyone comes across something they've never seen before or something they are unsure about on a regular basis. Don't be afraid to ask for help from a colleague, technologist, or radiologist.
- Always keep learning.

Afterword

We have reached the conclusion of this journey, one that has taken us from the very basics of ultrasound technique through to more challenging interventional and cardiovascular applications. We are conscious that this book is far from comprehensive in its scope. Many more advanced applications of ultrasound were not included here because we felt they were beyond the "basics" and these may form the subject matter of a future text. If after the first read, the content of this book seems overwhelming, we recommend re-reading the chapters at a slower pace and interspersing this with actual practice of the techniques and skills outlined. We have designed this book as a reference guide to allow you to pick up the skills gradually and at a pace you find comfortable. Your journey to the peaks of ultrasound mastery however, has only just begun and this text has led you merely through the foothills of this journey. Much of what remains lies in the realm of practice and you should take every such opportunity offered by both patients and willing volunteers. The great news is that the goal and the destination promise to be worth the effort. When teaching ultrasound skills to students and physicians, we are constantly rewarded by the great enthusiasm and excitement we encounter. I think one of the reasons why people are so excited about bedside ultrasound is that its future has yet to be written. They see its huge potential and it's out there for the taking. They understand that developing probe-handling skills today will enable them to practice better medicine tomorrow and it is this hope for our patients that will spur us all on to this end.

For further resources and more tips and tricks check out our website at www.figbus.net.

List of abbreviations used in this book

4CH	Apical four chamber view
2CH	Apical two chamber view
3CH	Apical three chamber view
AC	Abdominal Circumference
AML	Angiomyolipoma
AP	Antero-Posterior
AV	Aortic Valve
BPD	Biparietal Diameter
CC	Cranio-Caudal
CBD	Common Bile Duct
CRL	Crown Rump Length
CT	Computed Tomography
CW	Continuous Wave Doppler
DVT	Deep Vein Thrombosis
EDD	Estimated Date of Delivery
EMR	Electronic Medical Record
FHR	Fetal Heart Rate
FL	Femur Length

GA	Gestational Age
HC	Head Circumference
ICU	Intensive Care Unit
IVC	Inferior Vena Cava
IVS	Interventricular Septum
LA	Left Atrium
LMP	Last Menstrual Period
LV	Left Ventricle
LVOT	Left Ventricular Outflow Tract
MRI	Magnetic Resonance Imaging
MSK	Musculoskeletal
MV	Mitral Valve
OB	Obstetrical
PACS	Picture Archive and Communications System
PLAX	Parasternal Long Axis View
PROM	Premature Rupture Of Membranes
PSAX	Parasternal Short Axis View
PW	Pulse Wave Doppler
PV	Per Vagina
RAP	Right Atrial Pressure
SDP	Single Deepest Pocket
TAPSE	Tricuspid Annular Plane Systolic Excursion
TGC	Time Gain Compensation
TV	Tricuspid Valve
WES	Wall Echo Shadow (collapsed gallbladder containing multiple gallstones)

Acknowledgements

Any book such as this cannot be produced in isolation. The authors would like to thank the following individuals for their help and support during the writing of this book: Ken Winnig (Regional Director for Diagnostics, Northern Health), Ashley Hughes, Sam Barnes, Krystie Frederick, Jacinthe Lebrun and Sherri Lyons (Toshiba Medical Division, Western Canada), Kevin Hansen (General Electric Medical Division, British Columbia). Debbie Anderson, Genevieve Penny (FriesenPress) and finally Shyr's family, Karenza, Victoria and Daniel for their unwavering support.

References

1. Lichtenstein, D. A., Meziere, G., Lascols, N., Biderman, P., Courret, J. P., Gepner, A., Goldstein, I., Tenoudji-Cohen, M. (2005). Ultrasound Diagnosis of Occult Pneumothorax. *Crit Care Med*, 33, 1231-1238.
2. Blaivas, M., Theodoro, D., Sierzenski, P. R. (2003). Elevated Intracranial Pressure Detected by Bedside Emergency Ultrasonography of the Optic Nerve Sheath. *Academic Emergency Medicine*, 10, 376-81.
3. Rudski, L. G., Lai, W. W., Afilalo, J., Hua, L., Handschumacher, M. D., Chandrasekaran, K., Solomon, S. D., Louie, E. K., Schiller, N. B. (2010). Guidelines for the Echocardiographic Assessment of the Right Heart in Adults: A Report from the American Society of Echocardiography. *J Am Soc Echocardiogr*, 23, 685-713.
4. Nagueh, S. F., Smiseth, O. A., Appleton, C. P., Byrd, B. F., Dokainish, H., Edvardsen, T., Flachskampf, F. A., Gillebert, T. C., Klein, A. L., Lancellotti, P., Marino, P., Oh, J. K., Popescu, B. A., Waggoner, A. D. (2016). Recommendations for the Evaluation of Left Ventricular Diastolic Function by Echocardiography: An Update from the American Society of Echocardiography and the European Association of Cardiovascular Imaging. *J Am Soc Echocardiogr*, 29, 277-314.

5. Seldinger, S. I., (1953). Catheter Replacement of the Needle in Percutaneous Arteriography; a New Technique. *Acta radiologica, 39* (5), 368-76.

About the Authors

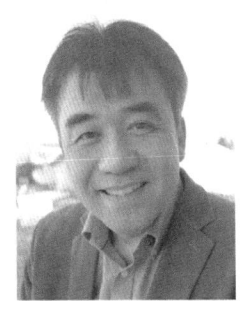

Shyr Chui is a radiologist with 20 years hands-on ultrasound experience. He obtained both his Bachelor of Arts and Medical Degrees at the University of Oxford before spending three years working in Internal Medicine and acquiring membership of the Royal College of Physicians. He completed residency training in Diagnostic Radiology at Guys and St Thomas' Hospital, London. He is currently practicing in Northern British Columbia, Canada.

Meagan Moi is a dual-trained general and cardiac sonographer with work experience in a hospital clinical setting for the past three years. She is a graduate of the British Columbia Institute of Technology with a diploma of Diagnostic Medical Sonography. Prior to her career as a sonographer, she obtained her Bachelor of Health Sciences from the University of Northern British Columbia.

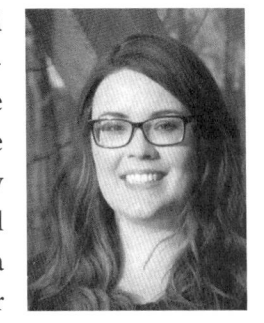

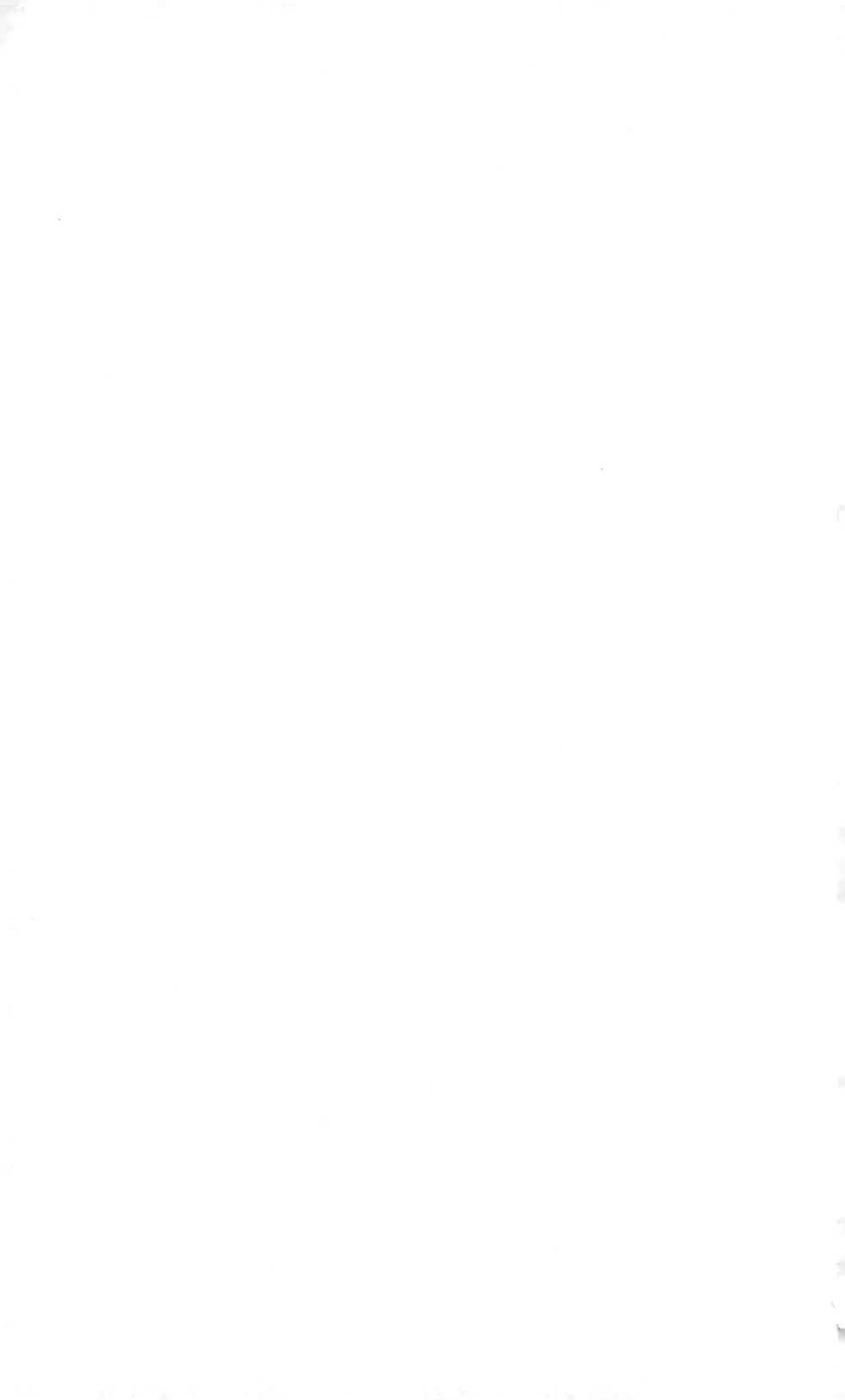

Printed in Canada